Student Workbook to Accompany

Administrative Procedures
Second Edition

Barbara Ramutkowski, RN, BSN
Pima Medical Institute, Tucson, Arizona

Kathryn A. Booth, RN, MS
Total Care Programming, Inc. & Wildwood Medical Clinic,
Henrico, North Carolina

Donna Jeanne Pugh, RN, BSN
Florida Metropolitan University, Jacksonville, Florida

Sharion K. Thompson, BS, AAB, RMA, CPT
Sanford Brown Institute, Middleburg Heights, Ohio

Leesa G. Whicker, BA, CMA
Central Piedmont Community College, Charlotte, North Carolina

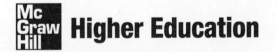

McGraw Hill **Higher Education**

Boston   Burr Ridge, IL   Dubuque, IA   Madison, WI   New York   San Francisco   St. Louis
Bangkok   Bogotá   Caracas   Kuala Lumpur   Lisbon   London   Madrid   Mexico City
Milan   Montreal   New Delhi   Santiago   Seoul   Singapore   Sydney   Taipei   Toronto

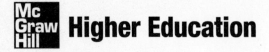

Mc Graw Hill Higher Education

STUDENT WORKBOOK TO ACCOMPANY ADMINISTRATIVE PROCEDURES, SECOND EDITION

6 7 8 9 0 CUS/CUS 0 9 8 7

ISBN-13: 978-0-07-297149-1
ISBN-10: 0-07-297149-5

Publisher, Career Education: *David T. Culverwell*
Senior Sponsoring Editor: *Roxan Kinsey*
Developmental Editor: *Patricia Forrest*
Editorial Coordinator: *Connie Kuhl*
Outside Developmental Services: *Julie Scardiglia*
Senior Marketing Manager: *James F. Connely*
Senior Project Manager: *Sheila M. Frank*
Senior Production Supervisor: *Laura Fuller*
Designer: *Laurie B. Janssen*
Compositor: *Interactive Composition Corporation*
Typeface: *10/12 Slimbach*
Printer: *Von Hoffmann Corporation*

Cover photo credits: Front (left to right); *Total Care Programming, Inc., Total Care Programming, Inc., Photodisc V18 Health & Medicine,* ' *Ed Bock/CORBIS,* ' *Royalty-Free/CORBIS, Photodisc: V40 Health & Medicine 2, Total Care Programming, Inc.*

www.mhhe.com

Contents

Preface

The *Student Workbook* provides you with an opportunity to review and master the concepts and skills introduced in your student textbook, *Administrative Procedures for Medical Assisting*, Second Edition. Chapter by chapter, the workbook provides the following:

Vocabulary Review, which tests your knowledge of key terms introduced in the chapter. Formats for these exercises include Matching, True or False, and Passage Completion.

Content Review, which tests your knowledge of key concepts introduced in the chapter. Formats for these exercises include Multiple Choice, Sentence Completion, and Short Answer.

Critical Thinking, which tests your understanding of key concepts introduced in the chapter. These questions require you to use higher-level thinking skills, such as comprehension, analysis, synthesis, and evaluation.

Applications, which provide opportunities to apply the concepts and skills introduced in the chapter. For example, using role play, you will perform such activities as developing a personal career plan and interviewing a medical specialist.

Case Studies, which provide opportunities to apply the concepts introduced in the chapter to lifelike situations you will encounter as a medical assistant. For example, you will have a chance to decide how to respond to a patient who calls the doctor's office to say that she is having difficulty breathing. You will also have an opportunity to practice taking and recording patient histories.

Procedure Competency Checklists, which enable you to monitor your mastery of the steps in the procedure(s) introduced in a chapter, such as Updating Medical Records.

Answers to the material in the *Student Workbook* are found in the *Instructor's Resource Binder*. Ask your instructor to let you check your work against these answers.

Together, your student textbook and the *Student Workbook* form a complete learning package. *Administrative Procedures for Medical Assisting*, Second Edition will prepare you to enter the medical assisting field with the front-office knowledge and skills necessary to become a useful resource to patients and a valued asset to employers and to the medical assisting profession.

Medical Assisting Second Edition Reviewers

Kaye Acton, CMA
Alamance Community College
Graham, NC

Jannie R. Adams, PhD, RN, MS-HSA, BSN
Clayton College and State University,
School of Technology
Morrow, GA

Cathy Kelley Arney, CMA, MLT (ASCP), AS
National College of Business and Technology
Bluefield, VA

Joseph Balabat, MD
Drake Schools
Astoria, NY

Marsha Benedict, CMA-A, MS, CPC
Baker College of Flint
Flint, MI

Michelle Buchman
Springfield College
Springfield, MO

Patricia Celani, CMA
ICM School of Business and Medical Careers
Pittsburgh, PA

Theresa Cyr, RN, BN, MS
Heald Business College
Honolulu, HI

Barbara Desch
San Joaquin Valley College
Visalia, CA

Herbert J. Feitelberg, BA, DPM
King's College
Charlotte, NC

Geri L. Finn
Remington College, Dallas Campus
Garland, TX

Kimberly L. Gibson, RN, DOE
Sanford Brown Institute
Middleburg Heights, OH

Barbara G. Gillespie, MS
San Diego & Grossmont Community College Districts
El Cajon, CA

Cindy Gordon, MBA, CMA
Baker College
Muskegon, MI

Mary Harmon
Med Tech College
Indianapolis, IN

Glenda H. Hatcher, BSN
Southwest Georgia Technical College
Thomasville, GA

Helen J. Hauser, RN, MSHA, RMA
Phoenix College
Phoenix, AZ

Christine E. Hetrick
Cittone Institute
Mt. Laurel, NJ

Beulah A. Hofmann, RN, MSN, CMA
Ivy Tech State College
Terre Haute, IN

Karen Jackson
Education America
Garland, TX

Latashia Y. D. Jones, LPN
CAPPS College, Montgomery Campus
Montgomery, AL

Donna D. Kyle-Brown, PhD, RMA
CAPPS College, Mobile Campus
Mobile, AL

Sharon McCaughrin
Ross Learning
Southfield, MI

Tanya Mercer, BS, RMA
Kaplan Higher Education Corporation
Roswell, GA

T. Michelle Moore-Roberts
CAPPS College, Montgomery Campus
Montgomery, AL

Linda Oprean
Applied Career Training
Manassas, VA

Julie Orloff, RMA, CMA, CPT, CPC
Ultrasound Diagnostic School
Miami, FL

Delores W. Orum, RMA
CAPPS College
Montgomery, AL

Katrina L. Poston, MA, RHE
Applied Career Training
Arlington, VA

Manuel Ramirez, MD
Texas School of Business
Friendswood, TX

Beatrice Salada, BAS, CMA
Davenport University
Lansing, MI

Melanie G. Sheffield, LPN
Capps Medical Institute
Pensacola, FL

Kristi Sopp, RMA
MTI College
Sacramento, CA

Carmen Stevens
Remington College, Fort Worth Campus
Fort Worth, TX

Deborah Sulkowski, BS, CMA
Pittsburgh Technical Institute
Oakdale, PA

Fred Valdes, MD
City College
Ft. Lauderdale, FL

Janice Vermiglio-Smith, RN, MS, PhD
Central Arizona College
Apache Junction, AZ

Erich M. Weldon, MICP, NREMT-P
Apollo College
Portland, Oregon

Terri D. Wyman, CMRS, CMS
Ultrasound Diagnostic School
Springfield, MA

Medical Assisting Second Edition Contributors

Kaye Acton, CMA
Alamance Community College
Graham, North Carolina

Jannie R. Adams, PhD, RN, MS-HSA, BSN
Clayton College and State University, School of Technology
Morrow, Georgia

Cathy Kelley Arney, CMA, MLT (ASCP), AS
National College of Business and Technology
Bluefield, Virginia

Russell E. Battiata
National School of Technology
Miami, Florida

Marti A. Burton, RN, BS
Canadian Valley Technology Center
El Reno, Oklahoma

Ann Coleman
Society of Nuclear Medicine
Reston, Virginia

Barbara G. Gillespie, MS
San Diego & Grossmont Community College Districts
El Cajon, California

Regina Hoffman, PhD
Midlands Technical College
Columbia, South Carolina

Donna D. Kyle-Brown, PhD, RMA
CAPPS College, Mobile Campus
Mobile, Alabama

Cynthia Newby, CPC
Chestnut Hill Enterprises, Inc.

Melanie G. Sheffield, LPN
Capps Medical Institute
Pensacola, Florida

Cynthia T. Vincent, MMS, PA-C
Wildwood Medical Clinic
Henrico, North Carolina

Terri D. Wyman, CMRS, CMS
Ultrasound Diagnostic School
Springfield, Massachusetts

CHAPTER 1

The Profession of Medical Assisting

REVIEW

Vocabulary Review

True or False

Decide whether each statement is true or false. In the space at the left, write T *for true or* F *for false. On the lines provided, rewrite the false statements to make them true.*

__T__ **1.** A practitioner is someone who practices a profession.

_____

__T__ **2.** The American Association of Medical Assistants works to raise standards of medical assisting to a professional level.

_____

__F__ **3.** You do not need to pass the American Medical Technologists certification examination to qualify as a Registered Medical Assistant (RMA).

You Do Need to Pass _____

__F__ **4.** A Certified Medical Assistant (CMA) credential is automatically renewed.

Every 5 years _____

__T__ **5.** Accreditation is the process by which programs are officially authorized.

_____

__F__ **6.** Externships are voluntary in accredited schools.

_____

__T__ **7.** A portfolio is a collection of your résumé, reference letters, and other documents that demonstrate your qualifications.

_____

__T__ **8.** The Medical Assistant Role Delineation Chart provides the basis for education and evaluation in the medical assistant field.

_____

Content Review
Multiple Choice

In the space provided, write the letter of the choice that best completes each statement or answers each question.

C 1. To receive certification or registration as a medical assistant, you must
   A. graduate from an approved program with a bachelor's degree in medical assisting.
   B. become a member of the American Association of Medical Assistants (AAMA) or American Medical Technologists (AMT).
   C. graduate from an approved medical assistant program and pass the AAMA or AMT examination.
   D. pass the AAMA or AMT examination.

C 2. Formal training programs in medical assisting
   A. are offered only at 2-year colleges.
   B. can be replaced by on-the-job training.
   C. must be approved by the AAMA or AMT.
   D. last 1 to 2 years and award a certificate, diploma, or associate degree.

B 3. Which of the following is clinical, not administrative, work?
   A. Greeting patients
   B. Preparing patients for examinations
   C. Creating and maintaining patient records
   D. Processing patient insurance claims

D 4. The definition of diplomacy is
   A. taking a stand about your beliefs and morals.
   B. a positive attitude.
   C. holding yourself to high standards.
   D. being able to communicate without offending anyone.

D 5. A person with integrity
   A. maintains high standards.
   B. is honest and dependable.
   C. is reliable.
   D. is all of the above.

Sentence Completion

In the space provided, write the word or phrase that best completes each sentence.

fast Growing 6. Medical assisting is a(n) _____ allied health profession because practitioners can handle many different duties.

Critical Thinking 7. Using _____ means evaluating circumstances, solving problems, and taking action.

Empathy 8. _____ is the ability to put yourself in someone else's shoes.

Flexability 9. The ability to change your schedule to adapt to coworkers' or employers' needs is called _____.

Communication 10. Effective _____ involves careful listening, observing, speaking, and writing.

Multi Skilled 11. A medical assistant who has learned different jobs and roles in all departments of a medical facility is considered to be _____.

Name _____ Class _____ Date _____

<u>ConServative Style</u> **12.** It is important that a medical assistant's appearance reflects a _____.

<u>Proffessional</u> **13.** Medical assistants should always conducts themselves in a _____.

<u>Integrity</u> **14.** Reporting a mistake to a physician is an example of _____.

<u>Diplomacy</u> **15.** Being able to understand both sides of any situation is an example of _____.

Short Answer

Write the answer to each question on the lines provided.

16. List three administrative duties performed by a medical assistant.

Greeting Patients
Handle Billing Bookeeping
Answering Phones.

17. List three clinical duties performed by a medical assistant.

Giving Injections
Sterilizing Medical Instruments
Draw Blood for testing

18. List three laboratory duties performed by a medical assistant.

Perform tests Such as Urine Pregnancy Test on Site
Collect, Prepare, and transmitted lab Specimens
Arranging Lab Services

19. Describe the goals of an annual employee evaluation.

_____
_____
_____

20. What rights are covered by Title VII of the 1964 Civil Rights Act?

You Have the right to Be free from any kind
of discrimination IN the workplace during Hiring
Process

21. List three areas of competence from the Medical Assistant Role Delineation Chart.

Administrative
Clinical
General or Trandisciplinary

22. List three areas that include the knowledge base of today's medical assistant.

General Medical knowledge
administrative knowledge
Clinical knowledge.

23. List three reasons why credentialing is important for a medical assistant's entry and advancement in the medical environment.

Malpractice

Managed Care Org

State and Federal Regulations

24. Why is a good attitude important in a medical environment?

Because you are working w/ People who are sick and Be understanding to what they are going Through.

25. What is tact?

_____

_____

_____

 Critical Thinking

Write the answer to each question on the lines provided.

1. Why should accreditation be based on a formal education program rather than on-the-job training?

_____

_____

_____

2. How might the size of an organization determine your responsibilities as a medical assistant?

_____

_____

_____

3. Why would someone who does not pay attention to details be poorly suited for a career as a medical assistant?

_____

_____

_____

4. Why is your appearance so important in health care?

_____

_____

_____

5. How can you determine if your attitude is what is required of a medical assistant?

_____

_____

_____

6. Give one example of integrity in the medical office.

_____

_____

_____

APPLICATION

Follow the directions for the application.

Appropriate Work Dress
Work with a partner to collect information on appropriate dress for work in a medical office.

a. Collect and request a collection of uniform catalogs from the Internet. Here are two popular sites: **www.Jascouniform.com** and **www.Allheart.com.**

b. Clip pictures of uniforms that you like and complete the "perfect" medical wardrobe.

c. Research and find pictures of clothing and accessories that are not suitable for the medical profession.

d. Make a collage of the two types of clothing—appropriate and inappropriate—and discuss with the class and instructor.

CASE STUDIES

Write your response to each case study on the lines provided.

Case 1

A patient calls just before your office closes to request an appointment. She's having difficulty breathing. You want to exhibit sound judgment. How will you respond?

_____

_____

_____

Case 2

Suppose you work as a medical assistant in a cardiologist's office. In your spare time, you read about new advances in heart medications. Even though only the doctor can prescribe medications, how might this knowledge help you in your job?

_____

_____

_____

Case 3

You are involved in a group interview. The medical assistant that you are interviewing is credentialed and has a lot of good experience. She seems pleasant but you notice that she has a "Right to Life" tattoo on her forearm, a tongue ring, and facial piercings. How do you think your elderly patients and female patients will perceive her? How might the physician perceive her?

_____

_____

_____

Name _____ Class _____ Date _____

Case 4

You have been assigned to work with a student extern. You notice that she gets upset whenever you correct her or try to show her something. She often arrives late for her assigned work time and cancels at least once a week. When she is there, you often have to find her, and she complains about tasks she doesn't like to do. What do you think her problem may be? Do you want to continue to work with her?

_____

_____

_____

CHAPTER 2

Types of Medical Practice

REVIEW

Vocabulary Review

Matching

Match the key terms in the right column with the definitions in the left column by placing the letter of each correct answer in the space provided.

__C__ 1. A physician who is a generalist and treats all types and ages of patients

__H__ 2. A physician who diagnoses and treats diseases of the nervous system

__A__ 3. A physician who specializes in the diagnosis and treatment of diseases of the heart and blood vessels

__N__ 4. To assess immediate medical needs of a patient

__I__ 5. A physician who specializes in treating patients with cancer

__J__ 6. A physician who diagnoses and treats diseases and disorders of the muscles and bones

__F__ 7. A physician who diagnoses and treats problems related to the internal organs

__G__ 8. A physician who studies, diagnoses, and treats kidney disease

__D__ 9. A physician who diagnoses and treats disorders of the gastrointestinal tract

__B__ 10. A physician who diagnoses and treats disorders of the endocrine system

__K__ 11. A physician who studies disease and the changes it produces in the cells, fluids, and processes of the entire body

__O__ 12. A physician who diagnoses and treats diseases of the kidney, bladder, and urinary system

__E__ 13. A physician who provides routine physical care of the female reproductive system

__M__ 14. A physician who performs the reconstruction, correction, or improvement of body structures

__L__ 15. A specialist who diagnoses and treats diseases and disorders with physical therapy

a. cardiologist
b. endocrinologist
c. family practitioner
d. gastroenterologist
e. gynecologist
f. internist
g. nephrologist
h. neurologist
i. oncologist
j. orthopedist
k. pathologist
l. physiatrist
m. plastic surgeon
n. triage
o. urologist
p. physician assistant
q. acupuncturist
r. massage therapist
s. chiropractor
t. doctor of osteopathy

Name _____ Class _____ Date _____

___T___ 16. A physician who uses a "whole person" approach to health care

___S___ 17. A specialist who treats patients who are ill or in pain without using drugs or surgery

___R___ 18. A specialist who uses pressure, kneading, stroking, vibration, and tapping to promote muscle and full-body relaxation

___Q___ 19. A specialist who uses a Chinese theory based on beliefs of how the body works

___P___ 20. A health-care provider who practices medicine under the supervision of a physician

True or False

Decide whether each statement is true or false. In the space at the left, write T for true or F for false. On the lines provided, rewrite the false statements to make them true.

___F___ 21. An endocrinologist diagnoses and treats physical reactions to substances such as dust and pollen.
   Studys Endocrine System

___T___ 22. An otorhinolaryngologist diagnoses and treats illnesses of the ear, nose, and throat.
   _____

___F___ 23. A neurologist uses medical instruments to correct deformities and treat external and internal injuries or disease.
   Surgeon

___F___ 24. A nephrologist uses medications to cause patients to lose sensation during surgery.
   IN Kidneys

___T___ 25. A doctor of osteopathy holds the title DO and focuses attention on the musculoskeletal system.
   _____

___F___ 26. A gynecologist specializes in the treatment of problems and diseases of older adults.
   Female Reproductive System

___F___ 27. A gastroenterologist specializes in the diagnosis and treatment of diseases of the skin, hair, and nails.
   Gastro Intestinal

___T___ 28. A pediatrician diagnoses and treats childhood diseases.
   _____

___F___ 29. A physiatrist specializes in taking and reading x-rays.
   _____

___F___ 30. A typical treatment plan for a chiropractor involves exercise programs, manual treatments, and anti-inflammatory medications.
   Uses NO Drugs or Surgery

___F___ 31. Massage therapists use techniques that increase circulation, remove waste products from injured tissues, and bring fresh blood and nutrients to areas of the body to speed healing.
   Kneeding, stroking, for full Body Relaxation

___F___ 32. Physician assistants are qualified to diagnose medical problems, order lab tests, and carry out treatment plans.
   only under Supervision of a Physcian

Content Review

Multiple Choice

In the space provided, write the letter of the choice that best completes each statement or answers each question.

B 1. A physician who wishes to specialize in a particular branch of medicine
    A. must complete 1 additional year of residency in that specialty.
    B. must complete an additional 2 to 6 years of residency in that specialty.
    C. must complete a bachelor's degree in that specialty.
    D. may do so without any additional education.

B 2. Radiology is the branch of medical science that
    A. is a subspecialty of neurology.
    B. uses x-rays and radioactive substances to diagnose and treat disease.
    C. provides the scientific foundation for all medical practice.
    D. studies and records the electrical activity of the brain.

D 3. A professional who has studied the chemical and physical qualities of drugs and dispenses such medication to the public is a
    A. nurse practitioner.
    B. pharmacy technician.
    C. medical technologist.
    D. pharmacist.

C 4. Which of the following takes health histories, performs physical examinations, conducts screening tests, and educates patients and families about disease prevention?
    A. Occupational therapist
    B. Associate degree nurse
    C. Independent nurse practitioner
    D. Licensed practical nurse

A 5. A health-care professional who works under the direction of a physician and manages medical emergencies that occur away from the medical setting is a(n)
    A. emergency medical technician.
    B. surgeon's assistant.
    C. radiation therapy technologist.
    D. pathologist's assistant.

Sentence Completion

In the space provided, write the word or phrase that best completes each sentence.

Family Practitioner 6. A physician who is a generalist and treats all types of patients is referred to as a(n) _____ by insurance companies.

Physical Therapist 7. Using therapy with electricity, heat, cold, ultrasound, massage, and exercise, a(n) _____ helps restore physical function and relieve pain following disease or injury.

Phlebotmist 8. _____ are allied health professionals trained to draw blood for diagnostic laboratory testing.

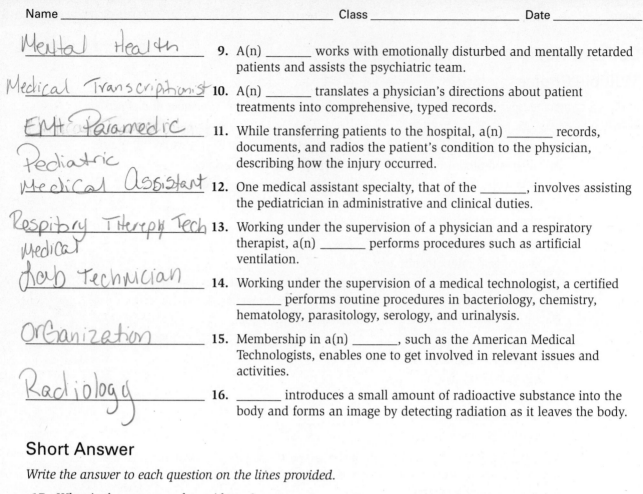

Mental Health   9. A(n) _____ works with emotionally disturbed and mentally retarded patients and assists the psychiatric team.

Medical Transcriptionist 10. A(n) _____ translates a physician's directions about patient treatments into comprehensive, typed records.

EMT Paramedic   11. While transferring patients to the hospital, a(n) _____ records, documents, and radios the patient's condition to the physician, describing how the injury occurred.

Pediatric Medical Assistant 12. One medical assistant specialty, that of the _____, involves assisting the pediatrician in administrative and clinical duties.

Respitory THerephy Tech 13. Working under the supervision of a physician and a respiratory therapist, a(n) _____ performs procedures such as artificial ventilation.

Medical Lab Technician 14. Working under the supervision of a medical technologist, a certified _____ performs routine procedures in bacteriology, chemistry, hematology, parasitology, serology, and urinalysis.

Organization   15. Membership in a(n) _____, such as the American Medical Technologists, enables one to get involved in relevant issues and activities.

Radiology   16. _____ introduces a small amount of radioactive substance into the body and forms an image by detecting radiation as it leaves the body.

Short Answer

Write the answer to each question on the lines provided.

17. What is the purpose of a residency?

So you Can Recieve Practical Training IN a Hospital-

18. When might a family practitioner send a patient to a specialist?

When patient Has a specific Condition ar Disease that requires advanced Care

19. What is the difference between a gynecologist and an obstetrician/gynecologist?

Gynecologist Performs Eams on Reproductive System ObGyn- Involves study of pregnancy, labor delivery and post pardem

20. What is the difference between an ophthalmologist and an optometrist?

Opthamologist Deals w/ eyes

21. What is the difference between a doctor of osteopathic medicine (DO) and a medical doctor (MD)?

DO- Practice Whole approach Treat Patient.
as a Whole Instead On Specific Systems.
MD- Generalist all Types and ages of Patients-

22. What are three duties of a medical secretary?

Maintaing Medical and admin files
assists Medical
Professional

23. In what types of settings can phlebotomists work?

medical Clinics
Labs
Hospitals

24. Explain the difference between a licensed practical nurse (LPN) and a registered nurse (RN).

LPN- Licensed Practial Nurse Can't perform all
Duties
RN- Graduated From Nursing Passes State Board.

25. What is osteopathic manipulative medicine? Formal Legal -Recognition By state

Helps Restore motion to these area's of Body
emproving function and Restoring Health

26. Describe the manual treatments and diagnostic testing that chiropractors use to treat patients.

Diagnostic Testing- X Rays - Muscle Testing
Manual Treatments Excersise Programs - Nutritional
advice.

27. Describe the principles of acupuncture.

Treats People w/ Pain Discomfort By
INSerting thin Hollow Needles under Skin.

Critical Thinking

Write the answer to each question on the lines provided.

1. What are the benefits of learning about the medical specialties and subspecialties?

_____
_____
_____

2. When specializing, what are the benefits of completing a formal 2- or 4-year training program rather than just learning on the job?

_____

_____

_____

3. List two allied health professionals with whom a medical assistant may work.

_____

_____

_____

4. Discuss how a medical assistant may interact with other health-care professionals or specialists.

_____

_____

_____

5. Why are patients referred to specialty physicians?

_____

_____

_____

APPLICATIONS

Follow the directions for each application.

1. **Career Plan**

   On a separate sheet of paper, develop a personal career plan using the guidelines below. Then share your plan with other students in the class.

   a. Record the current level of education you plan to pursue (for example, technical training program, associate degree, bachelor's degree). Also include the job title you would like to hold upon completion of that training.

   b. Write down the medical specialty areas that interest you. Decide which ones, if any, you might seek training in during the next 5 years, and underline those specialties.

   c. Research the kinds of additional training or education required for the specialties you selected. Next to each specialty, note the approximate time needed to complete the required training and education.

   d. If you do not plan to pursue a specialty, indicate when in the future you might reevaluate your decision and what factors might influence it.

   e. Present your career plan in the following format. Write the numbers 1 through 5 vertically down the page. Number 1 represents the current year, number 2 the next year, and so on. Indicate the career-related activity you plan to pursue next to the appropriate numbered year. Be as realistic as possible. For example, if you will attend school part-time while you work, allow a reasonable length of time to complete your education. Include career networking, job searching, continuing education, and joining professional associations, as applicable.

   f. After you have completed your career plan, share it with two classmates. Ask for their feedback, and incorporate their suggestions that will help you meet your goals. Repeat this process with two or more other classmates.

2. Specialist Interview

As a follow-up to studying the various specialties, choose a medical specialist to interview, and report on your findings.

a. Review the specialty careers described in the text. Select one.

b. Check the telephone book or other sources to find specialists in the area you chose. Write down the names and phone numbers of three to five specialists.

c. Call the offices of the specialists until you find a specialist who will grant you a 15- to 30-minute interview. Make an appointment for the interview.

d. Prepare a list of six to ten interview questions. Include questions that address the type and amount of education required, responsibilities and duties, and advantages and disadvantages of the specialty. Also include a question about what personal skills are required. Conclude by asking for advice that the specialist can offer someone interested in pursuing the specialty.

e. Dress professionally for the interview. Take your list of questions, a pen, and a pad to the interview.

f. Conduct the interview, keeping it within the time limit you promised. Thank the specialist for her time.

g. Send a thank-you note to the specialist within a week of the interview.

h. Share your findings with your classmates through a format of your choice: oral presentation, written report, or interview "question and answer" news article.

3. Medical Specialties

Research the Internet for specialties in which a medical assistant may be employed. Research the credentials needed and the experience required for the job. Then find a position within the specialty, and research what duties are performed by the position and how you may gain those skills. Report your findings to the class.

CASE STUDIES

Write your response to each case study on the lines provided.

Case 1

During a job interview, the staff administrator asks your opinion of professional medical associations. As a member of the American Medical Technologists, you explain the benefits of joining such an association. Describe these benefits below.

_____

_____

_____

Case 2

Suppose you have decided to become a urologist. List the steps you will need to take to reach your goal.

_____

_____

_____

Case 3

Your friend, who is also a medical assistant, wants to specialize as a surgeon's assistant. From your personal contact with her, you know she is disorganized and becomes excited easily, especially in high-pressure situations. What advice, if any, will you give her?

_____

_____

_____

Case 4

You are working as a lab assistant in a reference lab. You would like to work as a phlebotomist, but you need certification in phlebotomy as a requirement of the job. How would you research phlebotomy certification? Whom should you contact?

_____

_____

_____

CHAPTER 3

Legal and Ethical Issues in Medical Practice, Including HIPAA

REVIEW
Vocabulary Review
Passage Completion

Study the key terms in the box. Use your textbook to find definitions of terms you do not understand.

abandonment	durable power of attorney	law	negligence
agent		law of agency	subpoena
arbitration	electronic transaction record	liable	tort
bioethics		living will	treatment, payment, and operations (TPO)
~~breach of contract~~	ethics	moral values	
civil law	felony	malpractice claims	Uniform Donor Card
crime	Health Insurance Portability and Accountability Act (HIPAA)	Notice of Privacy Practices	use
disclosure			

In the space provided, complete the following passage, using some of the terms from the box. You may change the form of a term to fit the meaning of the sentence.

Medical workers must follow (1) _____ that govern the practice of medicine to prevent patients from filing (2) _____. Patients might charge (3) _____ if a medical worker does not perform an essential action or performs an improper one. A medical worker who stops care without providing an equally qualified substitute can be charged with (4) _____.

Doctors and their patients have an implied contract. A violation of that contract is a(n) (5) _____. If such a violation leads to harm, the violation is called a(n) (6) _____. Some lawsuits go to trial, whereas others are settled through (7) _____. If a case goes to trial, the people involved will receive (8) _____, requiring their presence in court.

According to the (9) _____, physicians are responsible, or (10) _____, for everything their employees do. A medical assistant is acting on the physician's behalf and is therefore a(n) (11) _____ of the physician.

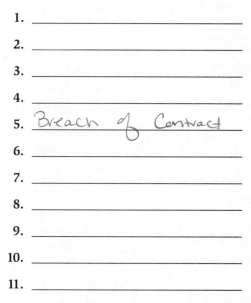

1. _____

2. _____

3. _____

4. _____

5. *Breach of Contract*

6. _____

7. _____

8. _____

9. _____

10. _____

11. _____

Medical assistants often assist patients in completing a(n) (12) _____, which states what type of treatment the patient wishes or does not wish to receive if the patient becomes terminally ill or permanently comatose. The patient may assign a(n) (13) _____ to a person who will make medical decisions if the patient cannot. People who wish to donate one or more organs upon their death, complete a legal document called a(n) (14) _____.

In addition to observing medical laws, medical workers must follow a code of (15) _____, which defines general principles of right and wrong. Medical workers may also have to deal with issues in (16) _____ when questions related to medical advances arise.

A(n) (17) _____ is an offense against the state. A(n) (18) _____ is defined as a rule of conduct. (19) _____ is considered a standard of behavior and the concept of right and wrong. (20) _____ serve as a basis for ethical conduct. Practicing medicine without a license is considered a(n) (21) _____. Crimes against the person are considered (22) _____.

HIPAA stands for (23) _____. Under HIPAA, (24) _____ limits the sharing of information within a covered entity, while (25) _____ restricts the sharing of information outside the entity holding the information. HIPAA will allow the provider to share patient information for (26) _____. The document under HIPAA that is the communication of patient rights is called (27) _____. The (28) _____ are the codes and formats used for the exchange of medical data under the HIPAA administrative simplification rule.

12. _____

13. _____

14. _____

15. _____

16. _____

17. _____

18. _____

19. _____

20. _____

21. _____

22. _____

23. _____

24. _____

25. _____

26. _____

27. _____

28. _____

Content Review

Multiple Choice

In the space provided, write the letter of the choice that best completes each statement or answers each question.

_____ 1. The term *res ipsa loquitur* refers to cases in which
   A. the patient has a previously existing condition.
   B. the doctor's mistake is clear to everyone.
   C. the patient has already filed a lawsuit.
   D. the doctor's error was caused by faulty record keeping.

_____ 2. If a physician decides to terminate his care of a patient, the physician must
   A. tell the patient face-to-face.
   B. send the patient a certified letter.
   C. obtain the patient's consent.
   D. inform the patient's family.

___D___ 3. Which of the following is *not* a legal procedure for medical assistants to perform?
   A. Maintaining licenses and accreditation
   B. Disposing of controlled substances in compliance with government regulations
   C. Determining needs for documentation and reporting
   D. Diagnosing a condition

_____ 4. A physician's receptionist asks patients to sign in and list the reason for their visit. This receptionist is violating the patients' right to
   A. confidentiality.
   B. a second opinion.
   C. sue for malpractice.
   D. be seen by the physician in a timely manner.

_____ 5. After disposable sharp equipment has been used, it should be
   A. recapped as soon as possible.
   B. wrapped in its original packaging.
   C. placed in an appropriate container.
   D. broken and placed in a wastepaper basket.

_____ 6. According to OSHA regulations, employee medical and exposure records must be kept on file
   A. for 5 years.
   B. during employment and 30 years afterward.
   C. until the employee leaves the job.
   D. until the physician retires.

_____ 7. Crimes such as attempted burglary and disturbing the peace are examples of
   A. felonies.
   B. misdemeanors.
   C. civil law.
   D. intentional crimes.

_____ 8. If a medical assistant gives a patient an injection after the patient refused the procedure, it could result in a charge of
   A. assault.
   B. battery.
   C. false imprisonment.
   D. *not applicable;* no charge would result because the physician ordered the procedure.

_____ 9. Preventing a patient from leaving the medical facility after administration of an allergy injection could be seen as
   A. an invasion of privacy.
   B. false imprisonment.
   C. an acceptable practice as long as it was documented in the chart.
   D. malpractice.

_____ 10. If a patient can prove that she felt "reasonable apprehension of bodily harm," it can result in what type of charge?
   A. Defamation of character
   B. Battery
   C. Assault
   D. Negligence

Sentence Completion

In the space provided, write the word or phrase that best completes each sentence.

_____ 11. Misfeasance refers to a lawful act that is done _____.

_____ 12. The four Ds of negligence are duty, derelict, _____, and damages.

_____ 13. The relationship between a doctor and a patient is called an implied _____.

_____ 14. Two types of infections that concern medical workers are the human immunodeficiency virus and the _____ virus.

_____ 15. Universal Precautions were developed by the Centers for Disease Control and Prevention to protect workers from exposure to _____ pathogens.

_____ 16. The most common kind of exposure accidents are _____.

_____ 17. _____, a division of the U.S. Department of Labor, requires employers to provide free training every year for employees who may be exposed to hazardous or infectious substances on the job.

_____ 18. Damaging a person's reputation by making public statements that are both false and malicious is considered _____.

_____ 19. Health-care practitioners who promise patients miracle cures or accept fees from patients while using mystical or spiritual powers to heal is considered _____.

_____ 20. A contract that is stated in written or spoken words is considered a(n) _____.

_____ 21. Torts that are committed without the intention to cause harm but are committed unreasonably or with a disregard for the consequences are _____.

_____ 22. A patient who rolls up her sleeve and offers her arm for an injection is entering into a(n) _____ contract.

_____ 23. A document that communicates patient rights under HIPAA is called _____.

Short Answer

Write the answer to each question on the lines provided.

24. What is the difference between malfeasance and nonfeasance?

_____

_____

_____

25. List eight types of personal information that is considered individually identifiable health information under HIPAA.

_____

_____

_____

26. What types of protected health information are subject to the privacy rule under HIPAA?

_____

_____

_____

27. HIPAA allows the provider to share what type of patient health-care information with outside entities?

_____

_____

_____

28. List five recommendations under HIPAA to ensure chart security.

_____

_____

_____

29. What are the civil penalties for HIPAA privacy violations?

_____

_____

_____

30. What is authorization under HIPAA?

_____

_____

_____

31. HIPAA allows patient information to be disclosed without authorization in special circumstances. List five entities with whom or situations in which patient information can be disclosed without authorization.

_____

_____

_____

32. Explain what a contract is.

_____

_____

_____

33. List and briefly define the four essential elements of a contract.

_____

_____

_____

Critical Thinking ━

Write the answer to each question on the lines provided.

1. A medical assistant promises a terminally ill patient a cure. Whom can the patient sue, the doctor or the medical assistant? Explain.

_____

_____

_____

2. Do you think the number of bioethical issues will increase or decrease in the future? Why?

_____

_____

_____

3. It may be possible that you will called to testify in a malpractice case for your medical facility or physician. It is important to conduct yourself in a manner that will help your physician's case. How do you think your courtroom conduct can help or hurt your physician's case?

_____

_____

_____

4. How can a medical assistant help prevent lawsuits?

_____

_____

_____

5. Documentation is an important aspect to malpractice suits. Name three chart entries that are important.

_____

_____

_____

6. How can a medical office safeguard protected health information that is transmitted via fax machines?

_____

_____

_____

APPLICATION

Follow the directions for the application.

Writing a Letter of Withdrawal

Work with two partners. Take turns being a medical assistant, a doctor, and an evaluator. Assume that the doctor has asked the medical assistant to write a letter of withdrawal to a patient.

a. The doctor should explain to the medical assistant what the problem with the patient is and why he has decided to withdraw from the case. The medical assistant should take notes and ask questions as necessary.

b. The medical assistant should then write the letter for the doctor. She should make clear the doctor's reason for withdrawing from the case. She should also include the doctor's recommendation that the patient seek medical care from another doctor as soon as possible.

c. After the foregoing tasks have been completed, the evaluator should critique the letter, keeping in mind the following questions: Does the letter include the doctor's reason for withdrawing from the case? Does the letter include the doctor's recommendation that the patient seek medical care elsewhere? Is the letter free of spelling, punctuation, and grammatical errors? Does it follow a business letter format?

d. The medical assistant and the doctor should discuss the evaluator's comments, noting the strengths and weaknesses of the letter.

e. Exchange roles and repeat the procedure with another student as a doctor who wishes to terminate care of a patient for a different reason.

f. Exchange roles again so that each member of the team has the opportunity to role-play the medical assistant, the doctor, and the evaluator.

CASE STUDIES

Write your response to each case study on the lines provided.

Case 1

A patient has a sexually transmitted disease but does not want you or the doctor to contact any former sex partners. The doctor has asked you to handle this case. How much can you do to make sure these people are notified?

_____

_____

_____

Case 2

A doctor is about to leave on a special family vacation for 2 months. A new patient comes to the office with a collection of unusual symptoms that do not seem to be serious. The doctor tells the patient to make another appointment for after his return from vacation so that he can order some tests. What kind of lawsuit is the doctor risking? What should the doctor do instead?

_____

_____

_____

Case 3

You work in a large medical office with three other medical assistants. One of the other assistants discusses her patients with you during your lunch break together. What, if anything, has the medical assistant done wrong? What should you do about it?

_____

_____

_____

Case 4

As you walk through the waiting room, a crying woman stops you. Her 14-year-old daughter is in an examining room. The daughter insisted on coming to the doctor but would not tell her mother why. The mother is afraid her daughter is pregnant or has contracted a sexually transmitted disease. What should you say to the mother?

_____

_____

_____

CHAPTER 4

Communication With Patients, Families, and Coworkers

REVIEW

Vocabulary Review

Matching

Match the key terms in the right column with the definitions in the left column by placing the letter of each correct answer in the space provided.

_____ 1. "You appear tense today."

_____ 2. "Please, go on."

_____ 3. Allowing the patient time to think without pressure.

_____ 4. "I follow what you said."

_____ 5. "Hi, Mr. Smith. Florida sure agrees with you."

_____ 6. "Can I help you with your shoes, Mrs. Adams?"

_____ 7. "Is there something you would like to talk about?"

_____ 8. "So, you are here today because of your swollen ankles and dizziness?"

_____ 9. "Describe your level of pain on a scale from one to five, with five being the most severe."

_____ 10. "Tell me when you feel anxious."

_____ 11. "So what you are saying is that you feel the most pressure when you exercise?"

_____ 12. Patient states: "Do you think this is serious enough to discuss with the doctor?" Medical assistant replies: "Do you think it is?"

_____ 13. "Your granddaughter's first birthday sounded wonderful. Now tell me more about your headaches."

_____ 14. "You're visiting the doctor today regarding a cough. How long have you been coughing?"

a. acceptance
b. offering self
c. making observations
d. reflecting
e. clarifying
f. exploring
g. offering general leads
h. giving broad openings
i. mirroring
j. recognizing
k. silence
l. summarizing
m. encouraging communication
n. focusing

Passage Completion

Study the key terms in the box. Use your textbook to find definitions of terms you do not understand.

active listening	conflict	passive listening
aggressive	empathy	personal space
assertive	feedback	rapport
body language	interpersonal skill	
closed posture	open posture	

In the space provided, complete the following passage, using some of the terms from the box. You may change the form of a term to fit the meaning of the sentence.

A medical assistant is a key communicator between the medical office and patients. When you make your patients feel at ease by being warm and friendly, you are demonstrating good (15) _____.

Communication with patients often requires (16) _____, which is evidence that the patient got and understood your message. Sometimes patients will give verbal confirmation. At other times, you will need to rely on nonverbal communication, or (17) _____. (18) _____ is a type of body language that conveys a patient's feeling of friendliness and receptiveness to your message. (19) _____ is a type of body language that conveys a patient's feeling of anger or lack of receptiveness to your message.

15. _____

16. _____

17. _____

18. _____

19. _____

True or False

Decide whether each statement is true or false. In the space at the left, write T for true or F for false. On the lines provided, rewrite the false statements to make them true.

_____ 20. Passive listening is the act of listening without the need for feedback.

_____

_____ 21. Active listening involves two-way communication in which the listener gives feedback or asks questions.

_____

_____ 22. Empathy is the process of identifying with someone else's feelings.

_____

_____ 23. An aggressive person tries to impose his position on others or tries to manipulate them.

_____

_____ 24. Rapport is a harmonious, positive relationship.

_____

_____ 25. Conflict in the workplace arises when two or more coworkers have the same opinions or ideas.

_____

_____ **26.** "The patient comes first" is a good definition of customer service.

_____

_____ **27.** Patients will often develop defense mechanisms to protect the mind from anxiety, guilt, and shame.

_____

_____ **28.** Patients will refer to hospice when seeking rehabilitation.

_____

Content Review

Multiple Choice

In the space provided, write the letter of the choice that best completes each statement or answers each question.

_____ **1.** Noise is anything that
  A. helps the patient give feedback.
  B. is a part of verbal communication.
  C. interferes with the communication process.
  D. is part of a communication circle.

_____ **2.** Positive communication with patients may involve
  A. getting them to limit their questions to save time.
  B. being attentive and encouraging them to ask questions.
  C. telling patients who ask questions that their concerns are foolish.
  D. allowing them to act on angry or abusive feelings.

_____ **3.** Which of the following is an example of negative communication?
  A. Maintaining eye contact
  B. Displaying open posture
  C. Listening carefully
  D. Mumbling

_____ **4.** Which of the following is *not* a communication skill?
  A. Active listening
  B. Anxiety
  C. Empathy
  D. Assertiveness

_____ **5.** When interacting with patients of other cultures or ethnic groups,
  A. assume that they have the same attitude toward modern medicine that you have.
  B. never involve other family members.
  C. never try to speak their language.
  D. never allow yourself to make value judgments.

Name _____ Class _____ Date _____

Sentence Completion

In the space provided, write the word or phrase that best completes each sentence.

_____ **6.** A communication circle involves a message, a source, and a(n) _____.

_____ **7.** Being _____ when communicating with patients shows them that you, the doctors, and other staff members care about them and their feelings.

_____ **8.** Your _____, which is the way you hold or move parts of your body, can send strong nonverbal messages.

_____ **9.** If a patient leans back or turns her head away when you lean forward, you may be invading her _____.

_____ **10.** Showing _____ for a patient can mean using a title of courtesy, such as Mr., or acknowledging his wishes without passing judgment.

_____ **11.** The _____ syndrome refers to the anxiety that some patients feel in a doctor's office or other health-care setting.

_____ **12.** Positive communication with superiors involves keeping them informed, asking questions, minimizing interruptions, and showing _____.

_____ **13.** A(n) _____ manual is a key written communication tool that covers all office policies and clinical procedures in the medical office.

_____ **14.** Explaining procedures to patients, expediting insurance referral requests, and creating a warm and reassuring environment are all examples of _____ in the physician office.

_____ **15.** _____, a well-known behaviorist, developed a human behavior model that states that human beings are motivated by unsatisfied needs.

_____ **16.** The ability to communicate with a patient in terms that she can understand, and making sure that the patient is comfortable and feels at ease is referred to as _____.

_____ **17.** A condition that results from prolonged periods of stress without relief is called _____.

_____ **18.** A world-renowned authority in death and dying, _____ developed a model of behavior that an individual will experience on learning of his condition. These behaviors are referred to as the stages of dying or the stages of grief.

_____ **19.** Obstacles that can interfere with your communication style are referred to as _____.

Short Answer

Write the answer to each question on the lines provided.

20. A health-care professional who speaks brusquely to patients is communicating negatively. What are three other examples of negative communication?

_____

_____

_____

21. What are four signs of anxiety?

_____

_____

_____

22. Cite five approaches that you can use to communicate with angry patients.

_____

_____

_____

23. What are three means of establishing good communication with a patient who is visually impaired?

_____

_____

_____

24. What are three things you can do to improve communication with a hearing-impaired patient?

_____

_____

_____

25. List four tips for communicating clearly with elderly patients.

_____

_____

_____

26. Describe three things you might do when dealing with very young patients.

_____

_____

_____

27. What are three rules for establishing positive communication with coworkers?

_____

_____

_____

28. List five examples of customer service in the medical office.

_____

_____

_____

29. List Elisabeth Kübler-Ross's five stages of death and dying and briefly describe them.

_____

_____

_____

30. List the five stages of burnout and describe some of the physical or personality changes that can occur with each stage.

_____

_____

_____

Critical Thinking

Write the answer to each question on the lines provided.

1. How does a person's body language convey his true feelings even when his words say otherwise?

_____

_____

_____

2. Explain how stress makes communication more difficult. Give an example in a health-care setting.

_____

_____

_____

3. Suppose a new medical office does not yet have a policy and procedures manual. What kinds of problems might arise?

_____

_____

_____

4. What therapeutic communication techniques can a medical assistant use when caring for an elderly patient? What defense mechanisms might elderly patients use?

_____

_____

_____

5. Explain how Elisabeth Kübler-Ross's model of the stages of death and dying can help both the families of terminally ill patients and the patients themselves.

_____

_____

_____

APPLICATIONS

Follow the directions for each application.

1. **Communicating With Patients**

   Work with three partners and role-play an interview with a patient. One partner should take the role of a patient, and one should take the role of a medical assistant who is communicating with the patient. The other two partners will act as observers. They should assign the patient an identity, such as an anxious elderly patient with a hearing impairment who is suffering from gout. The student playing the role of the medical assistant should be assigned three ineffective communication techniques. The observers should also determine a situation for the communication, such as a pre- or postexamination interview.

   a. The medical assistant and patient should assume their roles, using verbal and body language to communicate. The medical assistant will use appropriate skills to gather necessary information.

   b. The observers should take note of the body language and skills used by both the patient and the medical assistant. They should consider whether the patient is behaving and using body language that correctly expresses the patient's identity. They should observe whether the medical assistant is responding appropriately.

   c. Following the role playing, observers should critique the role playing of the patient and medical assistant. The observers should evaluate whether the body language and responses of the patient were realistic given the patient's identity and condition. They should evaluate whether the medical assistant used effective communication skills in reaching out to the patient. The observers should provide feedback about ways that the skills were appropriate and ways that they could be improved.

   d. The observers should identify each ineffective communication technique used by the medical assistant. The observers should provide feedback in correcting ineffective communication techniques.

   e. Exchange parts, create a new patient identity and situation, and repeat the role playing. Continue exchanging roles until each member of the team has had an opportunity to perform as observer, patient, and medical assistant.

2. **Policy and Procedures Manual: Writing Policies**

   Work with two partners as a team that is writing the policies for a new office policy and procedures manual. Assume that the manual will be organized in a loose-leaf notebook.

   a. As a team, talk about the topics that should be included in the manual. Have one partner take notes. Working together, decide which major policy areas your manual will cover, and create an outline.

   b. One of you should take the role of medical assistant, another should assume the role of office manager, and the third partner should act as the observer and evaluator. The medical assistant should choose one policy area from your outline. After discussing the policy with the office manager, the medical assistant writes a few sentences describing the policy. Scientific or medical journals, textbooks, or other sources may be used as references.

   c. After the policy is completed, the evaluator should critique it. In formulating feedback, the evaluator should consider these questions: Is the writing clear and concise? Is the policy described in enough detail? Will the policy help in the day-to-day workings of an office?

   d. The medical assistant and the office manager should discuss the evaluator's comments, noting the strengths and weaknesses of the policy as written.

   e. Exchange roles and repeat, choosing a different policy area from your outline.

   f. Exchange roles again so that each member of the team has an opportunity to write and evaluate a policy for the manual.

3. Burnout Test

Unmanaged stress can often lead to job burnout in the profession of medical assisting. Answer the following questions *true* or *false* and check your score to see if you are likely to become a victim of burnout.

_____ 1. I feel that the people I know who are in authority are no better than I am.

_____ 2. Once I start a job I have no peace until I finish it.

_____ 3. I like to tell people exactly what I think.

_____ 4. Although many people are overly conscious of feelings, I like to deal only with the facts.

_____ 5. I worry about business and financial matters.

_____ 6. I often have anxiety about something or someone.

_____ 7. I sometimes become so preoccupied by a thought that I cannot get it out of my mind.

_____ 8. I find it difficult to go to bed or to sleep because of the thoughts that bother me.

_____ 9. I have periods in which I cannot sit or lie down; I need to be doing something.

_____ 10. My mind is often occupied by thoughts about what I have done wrong or not completed.

_____ 11. My concentration is not what it used to be.

_____ 12. My personal appearance is not what it used to be.

_____ 13. I feel irritated when I see another person's messy desk or cluttered room.

_____ 14. I am more comfortable in a neat, clean, and orderly room than in a messy one.

_____ 15. I cannot get through a day or a week without a schedule or a list of jobs to do.

_____ 16. I believe that the person who works the hardest and longest deserves to get ahead.

_____ 17. If my job/school/family responsibilities demand(s) more time, I will cut out pleasurable activities to see that it gets done.

_____ 18. My conscience often bothers me about things I have done in the past.

_____ 19. There are things that I have done that would embarrass me greatly if they become public knowledge.

_____ 20. I feel uncomfortable unless I get the highest grade.

_____ 21. It is my view that many people become confused because they do not bother to find out all the facts.

_____ 22. I frequently feel angry without knowing what or who is bothering me.

_____ 23. I can't stand to have my checkbook or financial matters out of balance.

_____ 24. I think that talking about feelings to others is a waste of time.

_____ 25. There are times when I become preoccupied with washing my hands or keeping things clean.

_____ 26. I always like to be in control of myself and to know as much as possible about things happening around me.

_____ 27. I have few or no close friends with whom I share warm feelings openly.

_____ 28. I feel that the more you can know about future events, the better off you will be.

_____ **29.** There are sins I have committed that I will never live down.

_____ **30.** I always avoid being late to a meeting or an appointment.

_____ **31.** I rarely give up until the job has been completely finished.

_____ **32.** I often expect things out of myself that no one else would ask.

_____ **33.** I sometimes worry about whether I was wrong or made a mistake.

_____ **34.** I would like others to see me as not having any faults.

_____ **35.** The groups and organizations I join have strict rules and regulations.

Adapted, with permission, from *The Workaholic and His Family* by Frank Minirth, published by Baker Book House. Provided courtesy of Sound Advice, 1994.

CASE STUDIES

Write your response to each case study on the lines provided.

Case 1

A patient is seated in the waiting room. She looks extremely anxious and distracted. She has no family or friends with her for support. As a medical assistant, what course of action should you take? Explain.

_____

_____

_____

Case 2

A young child is about to receive an injection. He is scared and tearful. You know the injection will hurt slightly, but you decide to put the child's mind at ease by telling him that it won't hurt a bit. Is this the best way to handle the situation? Explain.

_____

_____

_____

Case 3

You are having a problem with a coworker. Both of you have the same job title and often work together to interview and prepare patients. This coworker cuts you off when you speak and contradicts you in front of patients. Her actions are affecting the way patients see you as a professional. How should you handle the situation?

_____

_____

_____

Procedure Competency Checklist

PROCEDURE 4.1   Communicating With the Anxious Patient

This procedure includes identifying the signs and sources of anxiety, using appropriate communication, and helping the patient recognize and cope with anxiety.

Complete the steps below. A scoring system has been provided for each procedure. The total score for each individual procedure is 100 points. Each step within the procedure is weighted according to the importance of that step and is noted in the column "Point Value." Steps that are of a more critical nature have been weighted with a higher point value. Record your point for each step in the column "Points Achieved."

Determine your mastery of each step in the procedure by assigning it a score of 1 to 4 in the last column: 1 = poor, 2 = fair, 3 = good, 4 = excellent.

On the basis of your scores, budget time for additional practice of specific steps.

Materials: None

Step	Point Value	Points Achieved	Mastery
1. Identify signs of anxiety in the patient.	10		
2. Acknowledge the patient's anxiety.	5		
3. Identify possible sources of anxiety, such as fear of a procedure or test result, along with supportive resources available to the patient, such as family members and friends.	10		
4. Do what you can to alleviate the patient's physical discomfort. For example, find a quiet place for the patient to wait, a comfortable chair, a drink of water, or access to the bathroom.	10		
5. Allow ample personal space for conversation.	10		
6. Create a climate of warmth, acceptance, and trust. a. Recognize and control your own anxiety. Your air of calm can decrease the patient's anxiety. b. Provide reassurance by demonstrating genuine care, respect, and empathy. c. Act confidently and dependably, maintaining truthfulness and confidentiality at all times.	10		
7. Using the appropriate communication skills, have the patient describe the experience that is causing anxiety, her thoughts about it, and her feelings. a. Maintain an open posture. b. Maintain eye contact, if culturally appropriate. c. Use active listening skills. d. Listen without interrupting.	15		
8. Do not belittle the patient's thoughts and feelings. This can increase anxiety.	5		

(continued)

Step	Point Value	Points Achieved	Mastery
9. Be empathic to the patient's concerns.	10		

10. Help the patient recognize and cope with the anxiety.
   a. Provide information. Helping patients understand their disease or the procedure they are about to undergo will help decrease their anxiety.
   b. Suggest coping behaviors, such as deep breathing or other relaxation exercises.
	10		

11. Notify the doctor of the patient's concerns.	5		

Time limit: 10 minutes   Add Points Achieved: _____

Observer's Name: _____

Steps that require more practice: _____

_____

Instructor comments: _____

_____

_____

CHAPTER 5

Using and Maintaining Office Equipment

REVIEW
Vocabulary Review
True or False

Decide whether each statement is true or false. In the space at the left, write T for true or F for false. On the lines provided, rewrite the false statements to make them true.

_____ 1. With a voice mail system, callers never receive a busy signal.

_____

_____ 2. Information stored on microfiche is full size.

_____

_____ 3. A warranty guarantees free service for the life of the product.

_____

_____ 4. A cover sheet provides information about a fax transmission.

_____

_____ 5. Leasing usually involves an initial charge and a monthly fee.

_____

_____ 6. You can hold microfilm up to the light to read it.

_____

_____ 7. Emergency repairs may be covered under a standard maintenance contract.

_____

_____ 8. A service contract is a list of tasks one is able to complete using a particular piece of equipment.

_____

_____ 9. Calling the supplier the minute a piece of equipment stops functioning properly is called troubleshooting.

_____

Content Review

Multiple Choice

In the space provided, write the letter of the choice that best completes each statement or answers each question.

_____ 1. An automated menu answering system
   A. answers calls and separates requests into categories.
   B. requires answering calls as they come in.
   C. does not notify the office when the caller presses the code for a patient emergency.
   D. is inappropriate for a medical office.

_____ 2. Answering services
   A. are unreliable
   B. are seldom used by medical practices.
   C. can have a direct connection to the doctor's office, answering calls after a certain number of rings.
   D. use mechanical voices rather than human voices.

_____ 3. A word processor is helpful to the medical assistant because
   A. corrections can be made easily within a document.
   B. documents can be stored in memory.
   C. the creation of correspondence is a function of the medical assistant.
   D. All of the above

_____ 4. Which feature is *not* available on a photocopier?
   A. Enlarging and reducing the size of a document
   B. Stapling
   C. Hole punching
   D. All are available.

_____ 5. Which statement is *not* true about fax machines?
   A. A fax machine uses a phone line.
   B. All fax machines require special thermal paper for printing.
   C. Faxes can be received 24 hours a day if the fax machine is turned on.
   D. When a fax has been successfully sent, most fax machines print a confirmation message.

_____ 6. What information can a medical assistant leave on a patient's telephone answering machine?
   A. Results of lab work
   B. Patient's new diagnosis
   C. Pregnancy test results
   D. A request for a return call

_____ 7. Interactive pagers are
   A. much like e-mail in nature.
   B. work in "real time."
   C. capable of talking to each other.
   D. All of the above
   E. None of the above

_____ 8. When the physician determines that a chart can be discarded, you should
   A. throw it in the trash.
   B. shred it.
   C. burn it.
   D. keep it for 7 years.

_____ 9. The postage meter

    A. is a convenient and cost-efficient way to apply postage to office correspondence and packages.

    B. functions only when there is money in the postal account.

    C. automatically senses the weight of a letter or package.

    D. A and B only

    E. All of the above

_____ 10. A leasing agreement for large office equipment is

    A. *always* preferable to buying.

    B. advantageous when you do not have enough money to buy the equipment but you need the service it provides.

    C. always less expensive over the long term.

    D. never price negotiable.

Sentence Completion

In the space provided, write the word or phrase that best completes each sentence.

_____ 11. When the office is closed, many practices use a(n) _____, which will answer the phone, take messages, and communicate them to the doctor on call.

_____ 12. When a physician is out of the office, she may carry a(n) _____ so she can be reached if needed.

_____ 13. Some fax machines print on specially treated paper, called _____, which reacts to heat and electricity.

_____ 14. A(n) _____ is a machine that applies postage to an envelope or package.

_____ 15. Medical assistants may be asked to _____ tape-recorded words into written text.

_____ 16. A(n) _____ imprints a check with the date, payee's name, and payment amount.

_____ 17. The only way to cancel an imprinted check is to _____ it.

_____ 18. If the price of the equipment or terms of the sale are not firm, there is room for _____, or bargaining for additional savings or more flexible terms.

_____ 19. A(n) _____ tells how a piece of equipment works, what its special features are, and how to troubleshoot problems.

_____ 20. Periodically, it will be necessary to conduct an equipment _____, which is a list of a business's equipment.

Short Answer

Write the answer to each question on the lines provided.

21. Explain how an automated menu telephone system works.

_____

_____

_____

22. What are the benefits of faxing a document?

_____

_____

_____

23. Compare the advantages and disadvantages of an electronic typewriter and a word processor.

_____

_____

_____

24. How might you post packages without a postal scale?

_____

_____

_____

25. Why is using a check writer safer than handwriting a check?

_____

_____

_____

26. List the steps involved in purchasing office equipment.

_____

_____

_____

27. Describe the basic contents of equipment manuals.

_____

_____

_____

28. What does a maintenance contract cover?

_____

_____

_____

29. List three steps in troubleshooting a problem with a piece of equipment.

_____

_____

_____

30. List three pieces of information that many medical practices keep about individual pieces of equipment.

_____

_____

_____

Critical Thinking

Write the answer to each question on the lines provided.

1. How does the almost instantaneous communication of information afforded by today's office equipment influence patient treatment?

   _____

   _____

   _____

2. Automated menus, voice mail, answering machines, and other office communication equipment reduce human contact between health-care workers and patients. What can you do to ensure that patients do not feel cut off by technology?

   _____

   _____

   _____

3. How does office automation affect the staff in a medical office and the care they give patients?

   _____

   _____

   _____

4. What could be a disadvantage of office automation?

   _____

   _____

   _____

5. What might be the advantage of building a relationship with one or two suppliers of office equipment rather than with many?

   _____

   _____

   _____

APPLICATIONS

Follow the directions for each application.

1. **Explaining How to Use Office Equipment**

   Work with two partners. One should take the role of a medical assistant who has worked in a medical practice for a while and knows how to operate all the office equipment. The second partner should take the role of a new medical assistant who is not familiar with the equipment. The third person should serve as an observer and evaluator.

   a. The observer should choose a piece of office equipment, such as a dictation-transcription machine. The experienced medical assistant should then give step-by-step directions on how to use the equipment. The new medical assistant should ask questions to clarify the directions.

   b. The evaluator should observe the training session while checking the directions given against those presented in the text.

   c. When the training session is complete, the evaluator should provide feedback by citing any omissions or errors in the instructions. All three partners should discuss the effectiveness of the session.

d. Now exchange roles. The new evaluator should choose another piece of equipment to describe in another round of training.

e. Exchange roles again so that each member of the team plays each role at least once. Repeat the activity until all partners achieve confidence in using each piece of equipment.

2. **Designing a Fax Cover Sheet**

Design a cover sheet to accompany a confidential faxed transmittal from a medical practice.

a. Decide on the type of medical practice. Create the names of the physicians and the address and phone number of the practice.

b. On an 8½- by 11-inch sheet of paper, decide what information to include. Then design your cover sheet.

c. Type the finished cover sheet. Check spelling, grammar, and punctuation.

d. Compare your cover sheet with those of other students. Decide whether you have provided all necessary information. Discuss whether cover sheets should be typed or handwritten and why.

CASE STUDIES

Write your response to each case study on the lines provided.

Case 1

You are the only one in the office. The physician calls and asks you to get a document over to the laboratory across the street. What can you do?

_____

_____

_____

Case 2

The office manager leaves you a note asking you to fax a document. You place the document in the sending tray of the machine and key in the phone number, but nothing happens. What do you do?

_____

_____

_____

Case 3

In researching a piece of equipment, you find two equally good options. One has a better price and one has a better maintenance agreement. How will you decide which to recommend?

_____

_____

_____

Case 4

You believe a word processor will help you work faster and more efficiently. Your coworkers say the office does not need a word processor. What should you do to convince them?

_____

_____

_____

PROCEDURE COMPETENCY CHECKLISTS

PROCEDURE 5.1   How to Use a Postage Meter

This procedure includes verifying funds available, applying postage to an envelope or label, and verifying the applied postage.

Complete the steps below. A scoring system has been provided for each procedure. The total score for each individual procedure is 100 points. Each step within the procedure is weighted according to the importance of that step and is noted in the column "Point Value." Steps that are of a more critical nature have been weighted with a higher point value. Record your points for each step in the column "Points Achieved."

Determine your mastery of each step in the procedure by assigning it a score of 1 to 4 in the last column: 1 = poor, 2 = fair, 3 = good, 4 = excellent.

On the basis of your scores, budget time for additional practice of specific steps.

Materials: Postage meter, addressed envelope or package, postal scale

Step	Point Value	Points Achieved	Mastery
1. Contact the company managing your account or the local post office to determine whether there are sufficient funds in your postal account.	10		
2. Verify the day's date. Check to make sure the postage meter is plugged in and switched on.	10		
3. Locate the area where the meter registers the date, and make sure the date is correct. If it is not, change the numbers to the correct date.	10		
4. Make sure all materials have been included in the envelope or package. Weigh the envelope or package on a postal scale to determine the amount of postage required.	10		
5. Key in the postage amount on the meter, and press the button to enter the amount.	10		
6. Check to see that the amount you typed is the correct amount.	20		
7. If you are applying postage to an envelope, hold it flat and right-side up. Seal the envelope (unless the meter seals it for you). Locate the plate or area through which the envelope can slide. Place the envelope on the left side, and give it a gentle push toward the right. Some models hold the envelope in a stationary position.	10		

(continued)

Step	Point Value	Points Achieved	Mastery
8. Create a postage label for a package. Follow the same procedure for a label as for an envelope. Affix the label to the package in the upper-right corner.	10		
9. Check to see that the printed postmark has the correct date and amount and that it is legible.	10		

Time limit: 10 minutes   Add Points Achieved: _____

Observer's Name: _____

Steps that require more practice: _____

_____

Instructor comments: _____

_____

_____

PROCEDURE 5.2 How to Use a Dictation-Transcription Machine

This procedure includes the mechanics of using the machine and proofreading and correcting the final document.

Complete the steps below. A scoring system has been provided for each procedure. The total score for each individual procedure is 100 points. Each step within the procedure is weighted according to the importance of that step and is noted in the column "Point Value." Steps that are of a more critical nature have been weighted with a higher point value. Record your points for each step in the column "Points Achieved."

Determine your mastery of each step in the procedure by assigning it a score of 1 to 4 in the last column: 1 = poor, 2 = fair, 3 = good, 4 = excellent.

On the basis of your scores, budget time for additional practice of specific steps.

Materials: Dictation-transcription machine; audiocassette or magnetic tape or disk with the recorded dictation; typewriter, word processor, or computer; blank paper or stationery; medical dictionary; regular dictionary; pen; correction fluid or tape (for the typewriter)

Step	Point Value	Points Achieved	Mastery
1. Insert the tape into the dictation-transcription machine. Turn on the typewriter, word processor, or computer.	10		
2. Place all materials, including a regular dictionary and a medical dictionary, within easy reach, and clear the area of items you will not use.	10		
3. Choose and insert the paper you will use. Set the margins and line spacing. Estimate the length using the scanning control.	15		
4. Press the foot pedal to start and stop the dictation-transcription machine.	10		

(continued)

Step	Point Value	Points Achieved	Mastery
5. To rewind the tape, use the reverse foot pedal.	10		
6. Pause the recording with the pause foot pedal, or stop it with the stop/start pedal.	10		
7. Adjust the speed and volume controls to help you work most efficiently.	10		
8. Proofread the final document, and make corrections directly on the document. Make sure the final document looks professional. Retype it if necessary. Proofread the final copy once again.	15		
9. When you have finished, turn off all the equipment.	10		

Time limit: 10 minutes   Add Points Achieved: _____

Observer's Name: _____

Steps that require more practice: _____

_____

Instructor comments: _____

_____

_____

CHAPTER **6**

Using Computers in the Office

REVIEW

Vocabulary Review

Matching

Match the key terms in the right column with the definitions in the left column by placing the letter of each correct answer in the space provided.

_____ 1. The physical components of a computer system

_____ 2. A blinking line on the computer screen showing where the next character that is keyed will appear

_____ 3. A device that is used to input printed matter and convert it into a format that can be read by a computer

_____ 4. The main circuit board that controls the other components in the computer system

_____ 5. A computer's temporary, programmable memory

_____ 6. A computer disk similar to an audio compact disc that stores huge amounts of data

_____ 7. Software that uses more than one medium—such as graphics, sound, and text—to convey information

_____ 8. A printout of information from a computer

_____ 9. A type of machine that forms characters using a series of dots created by tiny drops of ink

_____ 10. A system that allows users to run two or more software programs simultaneously

_____ 11. A collection of records created and stored on a computer

_____ 12. A method of sending and receiving messages through a network

_____ 13. A global network of computers

_____ 14. A software package that automatically changes the computer monitor at short intervals or shows moving images to prevent burn-in

a. CD-ROM
b. cursor
c. database
d. electronic mail
e. hard copy
f. hardware
g. ink-jet printer
h. Internet
i. motherboard
j. multimedia
k. multitasking
l. random-access memory (RAM)
m. scanner
n. screen saver

True or False

Decide whether each statement is true or false. In the space at the left, write T *for true or* F *for false. On the lines provided, rewrite the false statements to make them true.*

_____ 15. It is important to back up computer files and store them properly.

_____ 16. Telemedicine refers to the use of telecommunications to transmit video images of patient information.

_____ 17. CD-R technology enables the computer to comprehend and interpret spoken words.

_____ 18. Read-only memory (ROM) can be read by the computer, but you cannot make changes to it.

_____ 19. Random-access memory (RAM) provides speed to the computer. The more RAM, the faster the computer will perform.

_____ 20. To relieve the symptoms of carpal tunnel syndrome, hands while typing should be lowered below the waist.

_____ 21. The software is where information is stored permanently for later retrieval.

_____ 22. The central processing unit (CPU) is also called a microprocessor.

_____ 23. The blinking line or cube on the computer screen showing where the next character that is keyed will appear is called the pointing device.

_____ 24. A scanner is helpful in a medical office because patient reports from another doctor, a hospital, or another outside source can easily be entered into the computer.

Content Review

Multiple Choice

In the space provided, write the letter of the choice that best completes each statement or answers each question.

_____ 1. Another name for a PC or personal computer is a
    A. minicomputer.
    B. mainframe.
    C. calculator.
    D. microcomputer.

_____ 2. A notebook computer
    A. is also called a laptop.
    B. is also called a palmtop.
    C. does not require software.
    D. uses a tower case.

_____ 3. The best computer is
    A. a mainframe.
    B. a microcomputer.
    C. the model best matched to the need of the user.
    D. a notebook.

_____ 4. The device that made today's computer possible is
    A. the abacus.
    B. the punch card.
    C. the vacuum tube.
    D. the micro chip.
    E. All of the above

_____ **5.** The keyboard is the most common input device. Other input devices include
    A. pointing devices.
    B. modems.
    C. software.
    D. *A* and *B*.

_____ **6.** The shorter name for a modulator-demodulator is a
    A. scanner.
    B. cursor.
    C. modem.
    D. touch pad.

_____ **7.** The most common type of pointing device is a
    A. trackball.
    B. scanner.
    C. mouse.
    D. keyboard.

_____ **8.** Notebooks can operate
    A. on an AC adapter.
    B. on battery power.
    C. *A* and *B*
    D. None of the above

_____ **9.** The type of computer used by the government and large institutions is a
    A. mainframe.
    B. miniframe.
    C. modframe.
    D. modem.

_____ **10.** The term *software* means
    A. portable hardware.
    B. a set of instructions or program that tells the computer what to do.
    C. the input device.
    D. the cursor.

_____ **11.** The term *hardware* means
    A. portable software.
    B. a set of instructions or program that tells the computer what to do.
    C. the input device.
    D. the physical components of a computer system.

_____ **12.** The most expensive type of scanner is a
    A. flatbed.
    B. single sheet.
    C. double sheet.
    D. handheld.

_____ **13.** CD-ROMs
    A. look like disks.
    B. store less information than floppy disks.
    C. store more information than floppy disks.
    D. are flexible.

_____ 14. RAM
  A. is temporary or programmable memory.
  B. is permanent memory.
  C. is read-only memory.
  D. provides the basic operating instructions that the computer needs to function.

_____ 15. Intel Pentium microprocessors
  A. come in many common speeds.
  B. do not have a motherboard.
  C. are measured in megahertz (MHz).
  D. *A* and *B*
  E. *A* and *C*

_____ 16. A computer monitor
  A. may look like a TV screen.
  B. contains tubes.
  C. varies in dot pitch—the higher the dot pitch, the higher the resolution.
  D. does not display current, active information.

_____ 17. Laser printers
  A. are high-resolution printers.
  B. use a technology similar to that of photocopiers.
  C. All of the above
  D. None of the above

_____ 18. DOS
  A. is an operating system.
  B. is the original operating system.
  C. requires typing certain commands.
  D. All of the above

_____ 19. A computer tutorial
  A. is a small program designed to give users an overall picture of the product and its functions.
  B. requires technical support to operate.
  C. is designed for the advanced computer user.
  D. is a manual.

_____ 20. A computer password
  A. helps protect computer files.
  B. can be shared by more than one employee performing the same functions.
  C. stores information.
  D. backs up computer files.

Sentence Completion

In the space provided, write the word or phrase that best completes each sentence.

_____ 21. In a network, a(n) _____ is used as a centralized storage location for shared information.

_____ 22. The four main functions of computer hardware are inputting data, processing data, _____ data, and outputting data.

_____ 23. Carpal tunnel syndrome is caused by _____ hand and finger motions.

_____ **24.** The speed at which a computer can process information depends on the type and speed of its _____.

_____ **25.** If a hard disk drive has 1 gigabyte of storage space, that is the same as having 1000 _____ of storage space.

_____ **26.** Word processing, database, and accounting software are examples of software that is written for a specific purpose, or _____.

_____ **27.** _____ is a common computer application that allows you to write letters and reports and to transcribe a physician's notes.

_____ **28.** Requiring a(n) _____ limits the computer users who can access files.

_____ **29.** A computer _____ can damage or destroy information stored on a hard drive.

_____ **30.** Some day _____ technology may eliminate the need to transcribe physicians' notes.

_____ **31.** _____ is a computer that is very small and light. It cannot perform all the functions of a notebook computer but can be useful for people who need to have a computer available while they are out of the office.

_____ **32.** To use a modem, you must have access to a _____.

_____ **33.** You would not find a printer icon in a system that uses _____.

_____ **34.** Users who access computer files can be identified with _____.

_____ **35.** Screen burn-in can occur on a monitor if _____.

Short Answer

Write the answer to each question on the lines provided.

36. Compare a mouse and a trackball.

_____

_____

_____

37. Give one advantage and one disadvantage of a fax modem.

_____

_____

_____

38. Compare a diskette and a CD-ROM.

_____

_____

_____

39. What is the advantage of a dot matrix printer over a laser printer?

_____

_____

_____

40. What are two advantages of a Windows operating system over a DOS system?

_____

_____

_____

41. Patient records are stored on the hard disk drive of a computer. What are three ways that you could give a copy of those records to a consulting physician?

_____

_____

_____

42. What are four kinds of medical information that you could find using the Internet?

_____

_____

_____

43. What are three sources of information you might turn to if you are having problems using a software program?

_____

_____

_____

44. How does a surge protector help maintain a computer system?

_____

_____

_____

45. What should you do to protect diskettes from damage?

_____

_____

_____

Critical Thinking

Write the answer to each question on the lines provided.

1. If a medical office can afford only one computer, what kind should it purchase? Explain your answer.

_____

_____

_____

2. Why might it be useful to add a fax modem to a computer system even though the medical office already has a regular fax machine?

_____

_____

_____

3. Why might it be a good idea to take a computer course at an adult school or community college every few years?

_____

_____

_____

4. When buying a computer system, why is it a good idea to purchase all components from one vendor?

_____

_____

_____

5. How might a large medical office benefit from adding CD-R technology to its computer system?

_____

_____

_____

APPLICATION

Follow the directions for the application.

Typing and Editing a Letter on the Computer

a. Open a new file on your word processing program and type the letter below.

November 4, 20—

Mr. Karl Cousin
24 Elm St.
Wilmington, NJ 12345

Dear Mr. Cousin:

I have been unable to reach you by phone, so I am writing to confirm your appointment for Wednesday, November 9, at 2:30 P.M. If you will be unable to keep this appointment, please call us immediately at 555–7890 to cancel it or to change your appointment time. If we do not hear from you by Tuesday, November 8, at 2:30 P.M., we will assume you will keep the appointment, and you will be charged for the visit.

Please remember that payment must be made at the time of your appointment unless you have made other arrangements with our office. Be sure to bring any pertinent insurance forms with you and give them to us. We appreciate your cooperation and look forward to seeing you at our office on November 9.

Sincerely,

Marty Miller
Office Manager

b. Print a hard copy of your letter. Then make these changes to the computer file:
   1. In the inside address, add the patient's middle name: *James.*
   2. Spell out the word *Street.*
   3. In the second paragraph, delete these words: *and give them to us.*
   4. Move the last sentence of the letter to the beginning of the second paragraph.
   5. Save the letter under this file name: *confirm.apt.*
   6. Print a hard copy of your revision of the letter.

c. Now open a new file, and write another letter that a medical office might send to a patient, a newly hired staff person, or a laboratory, hospital, or consulting physician.

1. Print a hard copy of your first draft.
2. Exchange letters with a partner, and suggest any changes that would improve his letter.
3. Use the computer function keys to improve your letter by adding, deleting, and moving information.
4. Print your final version.

CASE STUDIES

Write your response to each case study on the lines provided.

Case 1

The medical office where you work has just begun converting to a computer system. The doctors are concerned about the confidentiality of the files. What will you recommend?

_____

_____

_____

Case 2

A coworker is intimidated by the office's new word processing program. Nearly every day she hands you a letter she has handwritten and begs you to enter it on the computer and print it so she can send it out. You are getting behind in your own work as a result. How can you solve this problem and still maintain a positive relationship with your coworker?

_____

_____

_____

Case 3

Recently it has become difficult to read information on the office's computer monitor. The faint image of one of the office form letters appears in the background. Explain how this problem might have been caused and what can be done to prevent it from happening to a computer monitor.

_____

_____

_____

Case 4

You enjoy painting with watercolors, but lately you have had trouble opening the paint containers and controlling the brush. A few months ago your office converted to a computerized record-keeping system. Explain a possible connection and how you would address this problem.

_____

_____

_____

Procedure Competency Checklist

PROCEDURE 6.1   Creating a Form Letter

This procedure includes entering, moving, and deleting text. Saving and printing the letter are also stressed.

Complete the steps below. A scoring system has been provided for each procedure. The total score for each individual procedure is 100 points. Each step within the procedure is weighted according to the importance of that step and is noted in the column "Point Value." Steps that are of a more critical nature have been weighted with a higher point value. Record your points for each step in the column "Points Achieved."

Determine your mastery of each step in the procedure by assigning it a score of 1 to 4 in the last column: 1 = poor, 2 = fair, 3 = good, 4 = excellent.

On the basis of your scores, budget time for additional practice of specific steps.

Materials: Computer equipped with a word processing program, printer, form letter to be input, 8½ × 11 paper

Step	Point Value	Points Achieved	Mastery
1. Turn on the computer. Select the word processing program.	20		
2. Use the keyboard to begin entering text into a new document.	20		
3. To edit text, press the arrow keys to move the cursor to the appropriate position to insert or delete characters, and enter the text. Use the "Insert" mode to add characters or the "Typeover" mode to replace characters.	10		
4. To delete text, position the cursor to the left of the characters to be deleted and press the "Delete" key. Alternatively, place the cursor to the right of the characters to be deleted and press the "Backspace" key.	10		
5. To move text, you must first highlight it. In most Windows-based programs, click the mouse at the beginning of the text to be highlighted. Holding down the left mouse button, drag it to the end of the block of text, and then release the button. Choose the button or command for cutting text. Then move the cursor to the place where you want to insert the text, and select the button or command for retrieving or pasting text.	15		

(continued)

Step	Point Value	Points Achieved	Mastery
6. Save your work every 15 minutes and at end of the task by choosing the "Save" command or button.	15		
7. Print the letter by using the "Print" command or button.	10		

Time limit: 10 minutes   Add Points Achieved: _____

Observer's Name: _____

Steps that require more practice: _____

_____

Instructor comments: _____

_____

_____

CHAPTER 7

Managing Correspondence and Mail

REVIEW

Vocabulary Review

Passage Completion

Study the key terms in the box. Use your textbook to find definitions of terms you do not understand.

annotate	editing	proofreading
clarity	full-block letter style	salutation
concise	identification line	simplified letter style
courtesy title	letterhead	
dateline	modified-block letter style	

In the space provided, complete the following passage, using some of the terms from the box. You may change the form of a term to fit the meaning of the sentence.

Most business letters are written on (1) _____ paper, which identifies the business. The (2) _____, which is placed about three lines below the preprinted letterhead text, gives the day, month, and year. In the inside address, the receiver's name usually includes a(n)(3) _____, such as Dr. or Mrs. The receiver's name is repeated in the (4) _____. In the (5) _____, or block style, all lines are flush left. In the (6) _____, the dateline, complimentary closing, and other parts of the letter begin at about the center of the page. The (7) _____ omits the salutation and the complimentary closing.

1. _____

2. _____

3. _____

4. _____

5. _____

6. _____

7. _____

True or False

Decide whether each statement is true or false. In the space at the left, write T for true or F for false. On the lines provided, rewrite the false statements to make them true.

_____ **8.** The letter writer's initials and the typist's initials appear in the notations.

_____

_____ **9.** Letters that are concise have unnecessary words and are vague.

_____

_____ **10.** A business letter that shows clarity can be understood easily.

_____

_____ 11. The editing process ensures that a document is clear, accurate, free of grammatical errors, organized logically, and written in an appropriate style.

_____

_____ 12. Proofreading means checking a document for errors before editing it.

_____

_____ 13. To annotate a document means to highlight key points or to add reminders, comments, or suggested actions in the margins or on self-adhesive notes.

_____

Content Review

Sentence Completion

In the space provided, write the word or phrase that best completes each sentence.

_____ 1. _____ refers to formal business stationary on which the doctor's (or office's) name and address are printed at the top.

_____ 2. _____ is used to mail or send large or bulky documents.

_____ 3. _____ is the most common envelope size used for correspondence.

_____ 4. _____ is used to send documents or materials, such as a slide, that may be damaged in the normal course of mail handling.

_____ 5. _____ paper is made from chemically treated wood pulp.

_____ 6. _____ refers to the look and feel of paper.

_____ 7. _____ type of paper has a rougher feel because it is embossed with a design, much like linen fabric.

_____ 8. _____ is a type of invoice or statement used to send an original bill.

_____ 9. _____ is a type of invoice or statement used to send a reminder when an account is 30 or more days past due.

_____ 10. _____ is typed two lines below the salutation and two lines above the body of the letter.

_____ 11. _____ is used when a letter is addressed to a company but sent to the attention of a particular individual.

_____ 12. _____ is a type of letter that is typed with all lines flush left.

_____ 13. _____ is a type of letter that is typed with the dateline, complimentary close, signature block, and notations aligned and beginning at the center of the page or slightly to the right.

_____ 14. _____ means that you say what you mean as briefly as possible.

_____ 15. _____ means that you state your message so that it can be understood easily.

_____ 16. _____ means to check a document for errors.

_____ 17. _____ should be used to look up the proper spelling of a medication.

_____ 18. _____ describes an error in involving the positioning of the various parts of a letter.

_____ 19. _____ must be placed in a certain location on the envelope for reading by the OCR.

_____ 20. _____ is the type of mail useful for heavier items that require quicker delivery than is available for fourth-class mail.

_____ 21. _____ is the type of mail that offers a guarantee that the item has been sent to the proper place.

_____ 22. _____ means to underline or highlight key points of a letter or to write reminders, comments, or suggested actions in the margins or on self-adhesive notes.

_____ 23. _____ is the action the post office will take when a piece of mail does not reach its destination.

_____ 24. _____ written on the outside of a letter or package means that the letter or package should not be opened by anyone but the addressee.

_____ 25. _____ is the process that ensures that a document is accurate, clear, and complete; free of grammatical errors; organized logically; and written in an appropriate style.

Short Answer

Write the answer to each question on the lines provided.

26. What are some advantages of learning to manage correspondence for a medical office in a professional manner?

_____

_____

_____

27. List three types of envelopes commonly used in a medical office, and briefly describe their uses.

_____

_____

_____

28. What is the difference between a modified-block letter style and a simplified letter style?

_____

_____

_____

29. Describe the voice of the sentence below. Then rewrite the sentence, changing the voice to make it more direct and concise.

The patient's blood sample was sent to you by our office on November 4, 1998.

_____

_____

_____

30. How do editing and proofreading differ?

_____

_____

_____

31. Why is an envelope with a typed address likely to be delivered more quickly than one with a handwritten address?

_____

_____

_____

32. Describe an accordion fold on a business letter, and explain why it is used.

_____

_____

_____

33. Describe a situation in which an item might be sent by fourth-class mail from a medical office.

_____

_____

_____

34. When processing incoming mail, why is it important to check the address on each letter or package?

_____

_____

_____

Critical Thinking

Write the answer to each question on the lines provided.

1. As an assistant in a new medical practice, what correspondence supply would you order first? Explain your answer.

_____

_____

_____

2. Briefly describe two types of letters from a health-care professional in which the tone should be formal and two types in which the tone could be relaxed.

_____

_____

_____

3. Which of these errors could be considered most serious: a formatting error, a data error, or a mechanical error? Explain your answer.

_____

_____

_____

4. Why should a medical assistant take the time to learn and use the rules of spelling, punctuation, and capitalization?

_____

_____

_____

5. What are three problems that could occur if a medical assistant handled incoming mail in a disorganized way?

_____

_____

_____

APPLICATIONS

Follow the directions for each application.

1. **Applying Basic Rules of Effective Writing**

   Read each of the following sentences for errors in spelling, word division, and capitalization and in the use of plurals, possessives, and numbers. If a sentence is incorrect, rewrite it correctly on the lines provided. Compare your corrections with those of a partner. Did you find the same errors? Did you miss any? Are there any writing rules that you need to study further?

   a. The Patients left oricle showed evidence of a recent infarktion.

   _____

   _____

   b. The abcess developed during the patients' recent trip to see his aunt.

   _____

   _____

   c. The patient was given a perscription for a 10-day supply of ilosone, a form of erythromycin.

   _____

   _____

   d. This 6-year-old patient reports falling from a slide at Ridge Street school this past tuesday.

   _____

   _____

   _____

   e. X-rays indicate hare-line fraktures of two cervical vertebra.

   _____

   _____

   f. Vigorous work outdoors in hot tempratures apparantly aggravated pastor Henrys heart condition.

   _____

   _____

2. Handling Incoming Mail

Assume that you are a medical assistant whose duties include processing incoming mail. Some of the procedures that you follow are described below. For procedures that are correct, write *correct* on the lines provided. For procedures that are incorrect, write the correct procedures on the lines provided.

a. Collect everything from the office mailbox, and process it a few items at a time throughout the day.

_____

_____

_____

b. In the top-priority pile, place letters and packages sent by overnight mail delivery, special delivery, registered mail, or certified mail. To this pile, also add any newspapers or magazines.

_____

_____

_____

c. After sorting the mail, open all the envelopes at once—except for those marked "personal" or "confidential"—and remove their contents, making sure to take everything out of each envelope.

_____

_____

_____

d. Throw away the envelopes as soon as you have removed their contents.

_____

_____

_____

e. Compare enclosure notations on each letter with the actual enclosures to make sure all items were included. Then make notes about missing items so that senders can be contacted.

_____

_____

_____

f. Staple each letter to its enclosures so they cannot become separated.

_____

_____

_____

g. Stamp any bills or statements with the date they are received.

_____

_____

_____

3. **Preparing a Business Letter**

Read the following case study:

You are a medical assistant working in a busy family practice office. One of the physicians says to you, "Please prepare a letter to go to Mr. Ford. He is the attorney for Mrs. Smith. Just check her chart to get his address. Tell him that Mrs. Smith has not been coming to her scheduled appointments. Tell him that I can't help her if she doesn't want my help!"

What questions might you have before you prepare this letter?

_____

_____

_____

_____

_____

_____

4. **Commonly Misspelled Words**

Correct the spelling of the following words.

a. _____ alltogether

b. _____ accquire

c. _____ unnesessory

d. _____ Wendsday

e. _____ dissapprove

f. _____ speciment

g. _____ Febuary

h. _____ comittee

i. _____ miscellanous

j. _____ truely

k. _____ menstation

CASE STUDIES

Write your response to each case study on the lines provided.

Case 1

A new coworker asks you to proofread a business letter that he wrote. You notice that the letter contains numerous formatting and mechanical errors. You also suspect that there may be data errors in the letter. What should you do?

_____

_____

_____

Case 2

You have just finished preparing several letters for signing by Dr. Morris, a physician in your office. Most of the letters need to be sent out today, but he will be extremely busy with patients for the rest of the day. Dr. Fuchs, another physician in your office, has authorized you to sign her letters. Should you sign Dr. Morris's letters and send them out right away? Explain your answer.

_____

_____

_____

Case 3

While opening the office mail, you discover that a patient has enclosed a check for more than she owes. Should you take a moment from processing the mail to call the patient? Why or why not?

_____

_____

_____

Case 4

A patient has come to your office without an appointment because he has unexpectedly run out of a prescription heart medication. The physician's schedule is completely full, so you cannot give the patient an appointment. However, you know that samples of this drug are in the sample cabinet. The patient should not skip any doses of this medication. What should you do?

_____

_____

_____

PROCEDURE COMPETENCY CHECKLISTS

PROCEDURE 7.1   Creating a Letter

This procedure outlines the proper method of formatting, editing, and proofreading a business letter.

Complete the steps below. A scoring system has been provided for each procedure. The total score for each individual procedure is 100 points. Each step within the procedure is weighted according to the importance of that step and is noted in the column "Point Value." Steps that are of a more critical nature have been weighted with a higher point value. Record your points for each step in the column "Points Achieved."

Determine your mastery of each step in the procedure by assigning it a score of 1 to 4 in the last column: 1 = poor, 2 = fair, 3 = good, 4 = excellent.

On the basis of your scores, budget time for additional practice of specific steps.

Materials: Word processor or personal computer, letterhead paper, dictionaries or other sources

Step	Point Value	Points Achieved	Mastery
1. Format the letter according to office procedures.	15		
2. Three lines below the letterhead, type the dateline.	5		

(continued)

Step	Point Value	Points Achieved	Mastery
3. Two lines below the dateline, type the special mailing instructions.	5		
4. Three lines below the special mailing instructions, begin the inside address.	5		
5. Two lines below the inside address, type the salutation.	5		
6. Two lines below the salutation, type the subject line.	5		
7. Two lines below the subject line, begin the body of the letter, single-spacing between lines and double-spacing between paragraphs.	5		
8. Two lines below the body of letter, type the complimentary closing.	5		
9. Leave three blank lines for the sender's signature; then type the sender's name and, below that, the sender's title.	5		
10. Two lines below the sender's title, type the identification line.	5		
11. One or two lines below the identification line, type the enclosure notation, if applicable.	5		
12. Two lines below the enclosure notation, type the courtesy copy notation, if applicable.	5		
13. Edit the letter.	15		
14. Proofread the letter.	15		

Time limit: 10 minutes   Add Points Achieved: _____

Observer's Name: _____

Steps that require more practice: _____

_____

Instructor comments: _____

_____

_____

PROCEDURE 7.2   Sorting and Opening Mail

This procedure includes verifying the addressee, sorting the mail according to priority, and reviewing incoming correspondence.

Complete the steps that follow. A scoring system has been provided for each procedure. The total score for each individual procedure is 100 points. Each step within the procedure is weighted according to the importance of that step and is noted in the column "Point Value." Steps that are of a more critical nature have been weighted with a higher point value. Record your points for each step in the column "Points Achieved."

Name _____ Class _____ Date _____

Determine your mastery of each step in the procedure by assigning it a score of 1 to 4 in the last column:
1 = poor, 2 = fair, 3 = good, 4 = excellent.

On the basis of your scores, budget time for additional practice of specific steps.

Materials: Letter opener, date and time stamp (manual or automatic), stapler, paper clips, adhesive notes

Step	Point Value	Points Achieved	Mastery
1. Check each address to make sure the letter or package belongs at your office.	5		
2. Sort the mail into piles, according to priority and type.	5		
3. Set aside all personal or confidential mail.	5		
4. Arrange all the envelopes with the flaps facing up and away from you.	5		
5. Tap the lower edge of the envelopes to shift the contents to the bottom.	5		
6. Open all the envelopes.	5		
7. Remove and unfold the contents of each envelope.	5		
8. Check each sender's name and address. If a letter has no return address, tape the address from the envelope to the letter. If the letter and envelope have different addresses, staple the envelope to the letter.	10		
9. Make sure the listed enclosures are included. If they are not, make a notation to contact the sender.	5		
10. Clip together each letter and its enclosures.	5		
11. Compare the date on each letter with the postmark date on its envelope. If there is a significant difference in the dates, keep the envelope.	10		
12. If no problems exist, discard the envelopes.	10		
13. Review bills and statements to make sure the amounts enclosed match the amounts on the statements.	10		
14. Stamp each piece of correspondence with the date of receipt.	15		

Time limit: 10 minutes   Add Points Achieved: _____

Observer's Name: _____

Steps that require more practice: _____

_____

Instructor comments: _____

_____

_____

CHAPTER 8

Managing Office Supplies

REVIEW

Vocabulary Review

True or False

Decide whether each statement is true or false. In the space at the left, write T *for true or* F *for false. On the lines provided, rewrite the false statements to make them true.*

_____ 1. Some mail-order supply vendors sell inventory kits, complete with cards and tabs or flags.

_____

_____ 2. When writing a check to a vendor to pay for an office order, it is correct to sign the physician's name on the check.

_____

_____ 3. When mailing a check to a vendor, it is important to mail the original order with the check.

_____

_____ 4. It is best to order supplies at the same time each week or month.

_____

_____ 5. Group buying pools provide savings only if everyone in the pool is ordering the same things.

_____

_____ 6. A vendor typically sends an invoice to the medical office, either to accompany the merchandise or separately.

_____

_____ 7. Keeping track of supplies involves creating supply lists and taking inventory.

_____

_____ 8. It is not important to maintain a working relationship with a vendor.

_____

_____ 9. Finding supplies is easier if you place large, bulky items at eye level and smaller items on lower or higher shelves.

_____

_____ 10. Chemicals, drugs, and solutions should be kept in a cool, dark place because light causes some substances to deteriorate.

_____

_____ **11.** To make the best use of space, you should stack items on the top shelf of the storage closet to the ceiling.

_____

_____ **12.** Material Safety Data Sheets are sometimes included with the item when ordered.

_____

_____ **13.** A good place to store the office's Christmas tree is in the back of the storage room near the air conditioner or furnace.

_____

_____ **14.** Medical assistants are responsible for ordering only medical supplies.

_____

_____ **15.** Durable items include pieces of equipment that may be used indefinitely.

_____

Passage Completion

Study the key terms in the box. Use your textbook to find definitions of terms you do not understand.

disbursement	invoice	rush order
durable item	purchase order	storage
efficiency	purchasing group	unit price
expendable item	reputable	wholesale price
inventory	requisition	

In the space provided, complete the following passage, using some of the terms from the box. You may change the form of a term to fit the meaning of the sentence.

As a medical assistant, your tasks may include ordering supplies for the office. To know which supplies to order, you must keep track of the office (16) _____. That is the list of supplies that your office uses and the amounts on hand. A good starting place is knowing about different kinds of supplies. Some supplies are (17) _____, so they can be used again and again. These items include telephones, computers, and stethoscopes. Other supplies, however, such as prescription pads, are (18) _____; they must be restocked as they are used.

By finding an item's (19) _____, you can tell exactly how much the office is paying per item. In some offices, supplies—no matter what the cost—cannot be ordered without a formal request from a staff member or a doctor. The form for this request is a(n) (20) _____. If you work at a group practice where doctors order different types of items, you may use a(n) (21) _____, which is a form that authorizes the practice to buy equipment and sometimes supplies. These forms usually are preprinted with numbers.

16. _____

17. _____

18. _____

19. _____

20. _____

21. _____

Many vendors would be glad to have your office's business. You can find a(n) (22) _____ vendor by looking for someone who fulfills orders correctly with quality items, delivers supplies in good condition, and charges a fair price. When the supplies arrive, the office will receive a(n) (23) _____— a bill from the vendor—and will pay for the supplies through a(n) (24) _____, or payment of funds. In some practices, you may order instead with a group buying pool, or with a(n) (25) _____, physicians who order supplies together.

By knowing how to manage supplies, you may be able to save your employer money. You will also demonstrate your own (26) _____, that is, your ability to get the desired result with the least effort, cost, and waste.

22. _____

23. _____

24. _____

25. _____

26. _____

Content Review

Multiple Choice

In the space provided, write the letter of the choice that best completes each statement or answers each question.

_____ 1. The best way to order office supplies is by
   A. telephone.
   B. fax.
   C. online.
   D. All of the above

_____ 2. If you find an error in a shipment, you should
   A. contact the vendor immediately so that the records can be corrected and missing supplies can be delivered immediately.
   B. make a note and make one call to the vendor each week.
   C. notify the physician.
   D. not be concerned because you can reorder the supplies.

_____ 3. When choosing a vendor, you should consider
   A. the quality of the products supplied.
   B. the company's reputation for service in the community.
   C. payment policies.
   D. All of the above

_____ 4. To determine the unit price on an item,
   A. divide the total price of the package by 2.
   B. divide the total price of the package by 3.
   C. divide the total price of the package by the quantity or number of items.
   D. None of the above

_____ 5. You should order by "Rush Order"
   A. routinely.
   B. on Fridays to avoid the weekend.
   C. only as absolutely required.
   D. on Mondays to compensate for the weekend.

_____ 6. Supplies should be stored in an organized and neat fashion
   A. because it is easier to clearly see when a supply is running low.
   B. because health regulations require that everything must be sterile.
   C. to prevent loss, theft, damage, or deterioration.
   D. *A* and *C*

_____ 7. When referring to office supplies, *expendable* means
   A. durable.
   B. items that are used and then restocked.
   C. clinical supplies.
   D. administrative supplies.

_____ 8. *Shelf life* refers to
   A. the age of the shelf where supplies are kept.
   B. the length of time after which the item is no longer usable.
   C. the length of the shelf on which the item must be stored.
   D. inventory.

_____ 9. Liquid soap and paper towels are examples of
   A. general supplies.
   B. clinical supplies.
   C. administrative supplies.
   D. noninventoried supplies.

_____ 10. When you receive a shipment, you should
   A. put it away immediately.
   B. record the date and the amount on the item's card or record page.
   C. notify the physician.
   D. notify the vendor that you have received the order.

Sentence Completion

In the space provided, write the word or phrase that best completes each sentence.

_____ 11. Vital supplies include items such as _____ and _____.

_____ 12. Nonvital supplies include items such as _____ and _____.

_____ 13. The proper way to store dated supplies is _____.

_____ 14. _____ are supplies that need to be ordered only occasionally.

_____ 15. _____ must be stored out of site and in a locked cabinet.

_____ 16. Lancets, iodine and betadine pads, sutures, and thermometer covers are examples of _____.

_____ 17. Appointment books, file folders, insurance forms, and paper clips are examples of _____.

_____ 18. Another name for a bill is a(n) _____.

_____ 19. _____ are usually bright, colored cards inserted directly into stock on the supply shelf to indicate when it is time to reorder an item.

_____ 20. _____ are groups of physicians who order supplies together to obtain a quantity discount.

Short Answer

Write the answer to each question on the lines provided.

21. What is the best plan for storing supplies in a small medical office?

   _____

   _____

   _____

22. What tasks are likely to be included in the medical assistant's responsibilities for maintaining supplies?

   _____

   _____

   _____

23. How does the size of an office affect the need for supplies?

   _____

   _____

   _____

24. Explain how inventory cards and colored adhesive flags can be used to track supplies that must be reordered.

   _____

   _____

   _____

25. Explain the function of reorder reminder cards.

   _____

   _____

   _____

26. Why is establishing a set time for ordering supplies important?

   _____

   _____

   _____

27. Briefly describe four categories of information you should obtain when investigating a vendor.

   _____

   _____

   _____

28. What procedure should you follow when receiving a supply shipment?

   _____

   _____

   _____

29. Why is ordering supplies important to a medical office?

_____

_____

_____

30. Why is wiser to order in bulk? Give an example.

_____

_____

_____

31. You notice that some items are always running out. What might you do to handle this situation?

_____

_____

_____

32. You suspect that an employee is taking office items home for personal use. What is the best thing to do?

_____

_____

_____

33. Why is it important to check an order carefully when it arrives?

_____

_____

_____

Critical Thinking

Write the answer to each question on the lines provided.

1. You have been put in charge of managing supplies for a large practice. You find that this responsibility takes most of your time. You would prefer to have more diverse duties. What might you do?

_____

_____

_____

2. The practice at which you work has been growing quickly. You think you may need to increase the quantity of certain items in the inventory, but you are not sure what quantity would be correct. What should you do?

_____

_____

_____

3. In the large office where you have started working, it has been the habit for most workers to keep their own stock of supplies at their various work areas. Why might you suggest that this system be changed?

_____

_____

_____

4. A new vendor offers you prices that are far below what you are now paying. You can save the office a great deal of money, but the brands are unknown to you. How should you handle the situation?

_____

_____

_____

5. As you check a shipment of supplies, you discover that there is a greater quantity of one item than was ordered and that one ordered item is missing altogether. What should you do?

_____

_____

_____

APPLICATIONS

Follow the directions for each application.

1. **Inventory Card or Page**

   You are setting up an inventory system for the office. Your first task is to design inventory pages to place in a binder. What information should you include for each item? List each category of needed information on the lines provided. Use a sheet of paper to design the inventory page.

   _____

   _____

   _____

2. **Unit Pricing**

   You are ordering 2-liter plastic bottles of saline solution for the office. Apex Medical Supply sells a ten-bottle package for $12.50. Acme Medical Supply sells the same brand and size in an eight-bottle package for $11.20. Which package is the better buy?

   _____

   _____

   _____

CASE STUDIES

Write your response to each case study on the lines provided.

Case 1

As the person at your office in charge of ordering supplies, you take a call from an unknown vendor. He tells you that he has an overstock of your brand of photocopier toner. He wants to get rid of it, so he will let you have it for half the regular price. He instructs you to send a check to a box number he gives you; then he will ship the toner to you. What should you do? Why?

_____

_____

_____

Case 2

Your office has used about ten boxes of no. 1 paper clips each month for the past 2 years. The size of the office staff and the office's patient load has stayed the same during that time. During the past 3 months, however, you have noticed that you are running out of the clips before you should. You start to notice that other supplies are running out more quickly than they should. How should you deal with the problem?

_____

_____

_____

Case 3

You receive a letter from a vendor threatening collection if an invoice that is now 6 months old is not paid immediately. You know that the invoice has been paid. How can you support your claim that your office has paid its bill?

_____

_____

_____

Case 4

As the new medical assistant at an office, you have been assigned the job of managing supplies. You review the supply-ordering system already in place. You research local supply vendors. Then you decide that the office would benefit by changing vendors for some of its clinical supplies. The doctor has been doing business with the present vendor for years and seems unwilling to change. Still, you ask for time to make a presentation to her and other members of the senior staff. What information should you present to make your case?

_____

_____

_____

PROCEDURE COMPETENCY CHECKLIST

PROCEDURE 8.1   Step-by-Step Overview of Inventory Procedures

This procedure includes establishing a needs list, devising a system, ordering, and verifying the receipt of as well as sending payment for office supplies.

Complete the steps that follow. A scoring system has been provided for each procedure. The total score for each individual procedure is 100 points. Each step within the procedure is weighted according to the importance of that step and is noted in the column "Point Value." Steps that are of a more critical nature have been weighted with a higher point value. Record your points for each step in the column "Points Achieved."

Determine your mastery of each step in the procedure by assigning it a score of 1 to 4 in the last column: 1 = poor, 2 = fair, 3 = good, 4 = excellent.

On the basis of your scores, budget time for additional practice of specific steps.

Name _____ Class _____ Date _____

Materials: Pen, paper file folders, vendor catalogs, index cards or loose-leaf binder and blank pages, reorder reminder cards, vendor order forms

Step	Point Value	Points Achieved	Mastery
1. Define with the physician the extent of your responsibility in managing supplies.	10		
2. Know what administrative and clinical supplies should be stocked in your office.	10		
3. Start a file containing a list of current vendors with copies of their catalogs.	5		
4. Create a want list of brands or products the office does not currently use but might like to try.	5		
5. Make a file for supply invoices and completed order forms.	5		
6. Devise an inventory system of index cards or loose-leaf pages for each item. Make sure that each card or page has all relevant data for the item.	5		
7. Have a system for flagging items that need to be ordered and those that are already on order.	10		
8. Establish with the physician a regular schedule for taking inventory.	5		
9. Order at the same times each week or month after inventory is taken, unless there is an unexpected shortage of an essential item.	10		
10. Follow ordering procedures that have been approved by the physician or office manager. Use the vendor's order form, type a letter of request, or order the supplies by telephone, fax, or e-mail to speed the process. Record the order information in the inventory file, and obtain an estimated order arrival time.	5		
11. When you receive the shipment, record the date and amount received on each item's inventory card or record page, and check the shipment against the order.	10		
12. Check the invoice against the original order and packing slip, and sign or stamp the invoice to show that the order was received.	5		

(continued)

Step	Point Value	Points Achieved	Mastery
13. Write a check to the vendor, have the physician sign it, and record the check number, date, and amount of payment on the invoice. Write the invoice number on the check.	10		
14. Mail the check and vendor's copy of the invoice to the vendor within 30 days, and file the office copy of the invoice with the original order and packing slip.	5		

Time limit: 10 minutes   Add Points Achieved: _____

Observer's Name: _____

Steps that require more practice: _____

_____

Instructor comments: _____

_____

_____

CHAPTER 9

Maintaining Patient Records

REVIEW

Vocabulary Review

True or False

Decide whether each statement is true or false. In the space at the left, write T for true or F for false. On the lines provided, rewrite the false statements to make them true.

_____ 1. A patient record, or chart, contains important data about a patient's medical history and present condition.

_____

_____ 2. Informed consent forms state that a patient has agreed to treatment.

_____

_____ 3. Documentation is the recording of information in the medical record.

_____

_____ 4. The problem-oriented medical record (POMR) system is a system of keeping charts that makes it easier to track a patient's progress by listing each problem separately.

_____

_____ 5. Signs are subjective conditions felt by the patient, such as pain or nausea, that cannot be seen or felt by the doctor or measured by an instrument.

_____

_____ 6. Symptoms are objective factors, such as blood pressure or swelling, that can be seen or felt by the doctor or measured by an instrument.

_____

_____ 7. SOAP is an approach to medical documentation in which information is recorded in patient records in the following order: subjective data, objective data, assessment, plan.

_____

_____ 8. Transcription is the transforming of written notes into accurate spoken form.

_____

_____ 9. A transfer of medical information involves giving that information to another party outside the physician's office.

_____

Content Review

Multiple Choice

In the space provided, write the letter of the choice that best completes each statement or answers each question.

_____ 1. When legal action is taken against a doctor, medical records can
   A. never be used in any way.
   B. support the doctor in defense against a claim.
   C. not be used to prove that an event or procedure took place.
   D. only be used to support a patient's claim of malpractice against a doctor.

_____ 2. Patient records are also valuable for
   A. patient education, evaluating quality of treatment, and research.
   B. patient education, research, and advertising for physicians' services.
   C. evaluating quality of treatment, patient satisfaction, and research.
   D. research, patient education, and compliance with government regulations.

_____ 3. Photocopies of patient information received by fax transmission on thermal paper should always be photocopied because
   A. a fax is not a legal document.
   B. a copy of the fax must be returned to verify that you have received it.
   C. fax copies made on thermal paper fade over time and may become unreadable.
   D. everything put in a patient's chart must be photocopied.

_____ 4. Which of the following is *not* a method for documenting patient information?
   A. Conventional, or source-oriented, approach
   B. POMR system
   C. Six Cs of charting
   D. SOAP documentation

_____ 5. All medical records are considered the property of the doctor, but no one can see a patient's records without
   A. the patient's oral consent.
   B. a court subpoena.
   C. the doctor's written consent.
   D. the patient's written consent.

_____ 6. Patient records are also known as
   A. patient research.
   B. patient forms.
   C. patient charts.
   D. None of the above

_____ 7. "Quality of treatment" refers to
   A. how appropriate and complete the medical care is.
   B. how expensive the medical care is.
   C. how many doctors have been consulted in the medical care.
   D. how much documentation there is in a patient record.

_____ 8. Which of the following information is described in informed consent forms?
   A. The outcome that might result with no treatment.
   B. The cost of a procedure.
   C. The details of every part of the procedure.
   D. All of the above

_____ 9. The first form used in initiating a patient record is the
    A. informed consent form.
    B. doctor's diagnosis form.
    C. doctor's treatment form.
    D. patient registration form.

_____ 10. Recording information in the medical record is called
    A. confirming.
    B. delivering.
    C. documenting.
    D. prescribing.

_____ 11. "Clarity" in charting means
    A. using the patient's exact words.
    B. dating all entries into a chart.
    C. not leaving out information.
    D. using precise descriptions and accepted medical terminology.

_____ 12. The information in a POMR (problem-oriented medical record) includes
    A. the database.
    B. the problem list.
    C. the educational, diagnostic, and treatment plan.
    D. progress notes.
    E. All of the above

_____ 13. The S in SOAP documentation stands for
    A. subjective.
    B. serious.
    C. sensitive.
    D. statistics.

_____ 14. The P in SOAP documentation stands for
    A. purpose.
    B. procedures.
    C. physical.
    D. plan.

_____ 15. The word that means "transforming spoken notes into accurate written form" is
    A. *subscription.*
    B. *prescription.*
    C. *transcription.*
    D. *recording.*

_____ 16. When speaking with an older patient,
    A. show an interest in the patient as a person.
    B. speak clearly.
    C. be patient.
    D. All of the above

_____ 17. What is the best example of the professional way to speak to an older patient?
    A. "You are not listening to me."
    B. "I can see how you might be confused. Let's see if I can help you."
    C. "Can you please hurry up?"
    D. "I am a little busy right now. Please call back later."

Sentence Completion

In the space provided, write the word or phrase that best completes each sentence.

_____ 18. The patient's past medical history, family medical history, and social and occupational history are included in a part of the chart called the _____.

_____ 19. It is important to date and _____ every entry you put in the patient chart so that it is easy to tell which items the medical assistant enters and which items other people enter.

_____ 20. When filling out patient charts, it is important to record patients' _____, not your interpretation of them.

_____ 21. To make chart data more concise, medical workers use standard medical abbreviations, such as "patient got _____" instead of "patient got out of bed."

_____ 22. All information in a patient's chart is _____, to protect the patient's privacy.

_____ 23. In a conventional, or source-oriented, record, all the patient's problems and treatments are recorded on the same form in _____ order.

_____ 24. In problem-oriented medical record keeping, each _____ is listed separately, making it easier for the physician to track a patient's progress.

_____ 25. When documenting problems, you must be careful to distinguish between signs, which are external factors that can be seen and measured, and symptoms, which are _____ that can be felt only by the patient.

_____ 26. Because the _____ of information in a patient's chart is important, check all information carefully before entering it.

_____ 27. The doctor's transcribed notes for the patient's chart should be initialed by the _____.

_____ 28. _____ provide physicians with easy access to patient information no matter where they are.

_____ 29. _____ charting describes a patient's condition by the use of four letters. The letters describe what the patient says, what the medical personnel see, an evaluation of the problem, and a directive for care.

_____ 30. _____ in medical records are not uncommon but must be changed immediately.

_____ 31. _____ means "to leave out."

_____ 32. _____ is the age at which most states consider an individual to be an adult.

_____ 33. To maintain patient _____, never discuss a patient's records, forward them to another office, fax them, or show them to anyone but the physician unless you have the patient's written permission to do so.

_____ 34. _____ contains a record of the patient's history, information from the initial interview with the patient, all findings and results from physical examinations, and any tests, x-rays, and other procedures.

_____ 35. In the _____, patient information is arranged according to who supplied the data—the patient, the doctor, a specialist, or someone else.

_____ 36. _____ means in the order of the date in which it occurred.

_____ 37. _____ means to be brief and to the point.

Short Answer

Write the answer to each question on the lines provided.

38. Explain the difference between patient signs and symptoms. List three examples of each.

_____

_____

_____

39. Describe the procedure for releasing patient medical records.

_____

_____

_____

40. List four additions that a physician might want to make to a patient's chart.

_____

_____

_____

41. List five tips for fast and accurate transcription of a doctor's recorded dictation.

_____

_____

_____

42. Describe the SOAP approach to medical record documentation.

_____

_____

_____

43. List the six Cs of charting.

_____

_____

_____

44. List six types of data contained in a patient's records.

_____

_____

_____

Critical Thinking

Write the answer to each question on the lines provided.

1. Why is it important to date every entry in the medical record?

   _____

   _____

   _____

2. Do you think the advantages of computerizing medical records outweigh the disadvantages? Explain.

   _____

   _____

   _____

3. What could be the danger in allowing medical workers to alter medical records at any time without question? Support your response with an example.

   _____

   _____

   _____

4. Why do medical records include notes of all telephone calls to and from a patient?

   _____

   _____

   _____

5. How do the rules of privacy for the release of a 15-year-old patient's medical records differ from the rules that apply to an 18-year-old's records?

   _____

   _____

   _____

APPLICATION

Follow the directions for the application.

Initiating a Patient Record

Work with two partners. Each of you should take turns being a medical assistant, a patient, and an observer/evaluator. Assume that this is the patient's first visit to the medical office.

a. Working together, create a model for a patient record. It must contain all the standard chart information, including forms for patient registration, patient medical history, and a physical examination. (You may use the forms shown in Figures 9-2 and 9-3 of the textbook as a guide.)

b. Have one partner play the role of the medical assistant and another partner play the role of a patient complaining of headaches. The third partner should act as the observer and evaluator. Have the medical assistant help the patient complete the patient registration form. Then have the medical assistant interview the patient and record the medical history, using standard abbreviations where appropriate, ending with a description of the patient's reason for the visit. The medical assistant should document any signs, symptoms, or other information the patient wishes to share.

c. Have the evaluator critique the interview and the documentation in the patient chart. The critique should take into account the accuracy of the documentation, the order in which the medical history was taken, and the history's completeness. The evaluator should also note the medical assistant's ability to follow the six Cs of charting, including the correct use of medical abbreviations.

d. The medical assistant, the patient, and the observer should discuss the observer's comments, noting the strengths and weaknesses of the interview and the quality of the documentation.

e. Exchange roles and repeat the exercise with a new patient. Allow the student playing the patient to choose a different medical problem.

f. Exchange roles again so that each member of the team has an opportunity to play the interviewer, the patient, and the observer once.

CASE STUDIES

Write your response to each case study on the lines provided.

Case 1

You accidentally throw out a sheet of a patient's medical chart. The trash has already been taken away, so there is no chance for you to get it back. You are new in the office, and you are afraid of losing your job if you tell the doctor what you have done. You remember the information that was on the sheet. You think you can easily rewrite it. What should you do?

_____

_____

_____

Case 2

The doctor you work for reads information about her patients into a tape recorder. You then must transcribe the information and enter it into patient charts. The doctor has a pronounced accent, and many of her words are difficult for you to understand. How should you handle the situation?

_____

_____

_____

Case 3

A former patient of the doctor you work for calls and asks you to send her medical records to her new doctor. She says it is important that the records get to her new doctor by this afternoon and asks you to fax them. Would you have a problem with this request? Why or why not?

_____

_____

_____

Case 4

Dr. Smith receives laboratory results from a test performed on Mr. Jones. He calls Mr. Jones at home on Monday, July 6, at 10:00 A.M. He gets no answer, but he leaves a message on Mr. Jones's answering machine asking him to call the office. By 10:00 A.M. the next morning, Dr. Smith has received no answer from Mr. Jones. He calls again and reaches Mrs. Jones and asks her to have her husband call the office. Mr. Jones calls the doctor's office at 2:30 that afternoon. Dr. Smith discusses the test results with Mr. Jones and asks him to make an appointment for the following week. Mr. Jones is connected with the receptionist. He makes an appointment for 11:00 A.M. on July 12. As a medical assistant, how would you record this series of events in Mr. Jones's chart?

_____

_____

_____

PROCEDURE COMPETENCY CHECKLISTS

PROCEDURE 9.1   Correcting Medical Records

This procedure outlines the steps to be taken to correct a medical record within medical legal boundaries.

Complete the steps below. A scoring system has been provided for each procedure. The total score for each individual procedure is 100 points. Each step within the procedure is weighted according to the importance of that step and is noted in the column "Point Value." Steps that are of a more critical nature have been weighted with a higher point value. Record your points for each step in the column "Points Achieved."

Determine your mastery of each step in the procedure by assigning it a score of 1 to 4 in the last column: 1 = poor, 2 = fair, 3 = good, 4 = excellent.

On the basis of your scores, budget time for additional practice of specific steps.

Materials: Patient file, other pertinent documents that contain the information to be used in making corrections (for example, transcribed notes, telephone notes, physician's comments, correspondence), a good ballpoint pen

Step	Point Value	Points Achieved	Mastery
1. Make the correction in a way that does not suggest any intention to deceive or cover up a lack of proper medical care.	20		
2. When deleting information, draw a line through the original information, but do not erase it or completely cover it up.	15		
3. Write or type in the correct information above or below the original line or in the margin. If you need to attach another sheet of paper with the correction on it, indicate in the record where the correction can be found.	15		
4. Place a note near the correction explaining why it was made. Never make any change without noting the reason for it.	15		

(continued)

Step	Point Value	Points Achieved	Mastery
5. Enter the date and time, and initial the correction.	20		
6. If possible, have the physician or another staff member witness and initial the correction.	15		

Time limit: 10 minutes   Add Points Achieved: _____

Observer's Name: _____

Steps that require more practice: _____

_____

Instructor comments: _____

_____

_____

PROCEDURE 9.2   Updating Medical Records

This procedure includes verifying the right record, transcribing the physician's notes, noting patient telephone communications, editing the entries, and filing the information in the patient's folder.

Complete the steps below. A scoring system has been provided for each procedure. The total score for each individual procedure is 100 points. Each step within the procedure is weighted according to the importance of that step and is noted in the column "Point Value." Steps that are of a more critical nature have been weighted with a higher point value. Record your points for each step in the column "Points Achieved."

Determine your mastery of each step in the procedure by assigning it a score of 1 to 4 in the last column: 1 = poor, 2 = fair, 3 = good, 4 = excellent.

On the basis of your scores, budget time for additional practice of specific steps.

Materials: Patient file, other pertinent documents (test results, x-rays, telephone notes, correspondence), good ballpoint pen, notebook, typewriter/transcribing equipment

Step	Point Value	Points Achieved	Mastery
1. Verify that you have the right records for the right patient.	15		
2. Transcribe dictated doctor's notes as soon as possible, and enter them into the patient record.	10		
3. Spell out names of disorders, diseases, medication, and other terms the first time you enter them, followed by the appropriate abbreviation (for example: congestive heart failure [CHF]). Thereafter, use the abbreviation.	15		
4. Enter only what the doctor has dictated. Date and initial each entry.	15		

(continued)

Step	Point Value	Points Achieved	Mastery
5. Ask the doctor where in the file to record laboratory test results. Follow his instructions, then date and initial each entry. Note in the chart the date of the test and the results.	5		
6. Make a note of all telephone calls to and from the patient. Date and initial the entries. These entries may also include the doctor's observations, changes in the patient's medications, and so on.	10		
7. Read over the entries for omissions or mistakes. Ask the doctor to answer any questions you have.	10		
8. Make sure you have dated and initialed each entry.	5		
9. Be sure all documents are included in the file.	10		
10. Replace the patient's file in the filing system as soon as possible.	5		

Time limit: 10 minutes   Add Points Achieved: _____

Observer's Name: _____

Steps that require more practice: _____

_____

Instructor comments: _____

_____

_____

CHAPTER 10

Managing the Office Medical Records

REVIEW

Vocabulary Review

Matching

Match the key terms in the right column with the definitions in the left column by placing the letter of each correct answer in the space provided.

_____ 1. Pullout drawers in which hanging file folders are hung

_____ 2. Horizontal filing cabinets

_____ 3. Reminder files

_____ 4. Frequently used files

_____ 5. Infrequently used files

_____ 6. Files that are no longer consulted

a. inactive files
b. vertical files
c. active files
d. tickler files
e. lateral files
f. closed files

True or False

Decide whether each statement is true or false. In the space at the left, write T *for true or* F *for false. On the lines provided, rewrite the false statements to make them true.*

_____ 7. One way to use color-coded filing is in conjunction with an alphabetic filing system.

_____

_____ 8. Someone in the office should be assigned the responsibility to check the tickler file.

_____

_____ 9. Some practices require that records be returned to the files as soon as they are no longer needed. In other practices, the timing is up to you.

_____

_____ 10. Paper files are not bulky to store.

_____

_____ 11. Physicians must permanently keep all immunization records on file in the office.

_____

_____ 12. Most legal consultants advise their clients to retain patient records for 3 years to avoid malpractice suits.

_____

_____ 13. Vertical file cabinets are also called lateral file cabinets.

_____

_____ 14. A records management system refers to the way patient records are created, filed, and maintained.

_____

_____ 15. Although you may never have to buy filing equipment, buying filing supplies may be one of your regular responsibilities as a medical assistant.

_____

_____ 16. The disadvantage of compactible files is that they take up more space than other types of filing cabinets.

_____

_____ 17. You should write the name of a patient on the tab of a file folder.

_____

_____ 18. Use a file guide as a placeholder to indicate that a file has been taken out of the filing system.

_____

_____ 19. Use an out guide as a placeholder to show that a file has been cross-referenced.

_____

_____ 20. All filing systems organize patient records in sequential order.

_____

_____ 21. In an alphabetic filing system, files are placed in alphabetic order according to the patients' first names.

_____

_____ 22. In a numeric filing system, files are organized according to numbers assigned to each patient.

_____

_____ 23. A file that has been cross-referenced has been placed in only one location.

_____

_____ 24. A retention schedule specifies how long to keep patient records in the office after the files have become inactive or closed.

_____

Content Review

Multiple Choice

In the space provided, write the letter of the choice that best completes each statement or answers each question.

_____ 1. An advantage of filing shelves over filing cabinets is that
   A. filing shelves can be compacted to conserve space.
   B. several people can work at filing shelves simultaneously.
   C. filing shelves are more secure.
   D. files can be found more easily.

_____ **2.** A numeric filing system
   A. is not used when patient confidentiality is especially important.
   B. organizes records according to the patient's last name.
   C. may include numbers that indicate where in the filing system a file can be found.
   D. is the only practical system for a large practice.

_____ **3.** Use color coding for files
   A. only when using a numeric filing system.
   B. to identify files belonging to specific categories of patients.
   C. whenever patient confidentiality is a significant issue.
   D. to reduce the risk of misplacing files.

_____ **4.** For tickler files to work effectively, they must be
   A. kept in file folders.
   B. located in a secure area.
   C. checked frequently.
   D. organized into weekly files.

_____ **5.** Compactible files are
   A. kept on rolling shelves that slide along permanent tracks in the floor.
   B. stored in a circular fashion.
   C. also called tubs.
   D. also called boxes.

_____ **6.** When files are labeled with the patient's last name first, followed by the first or given name and then the middle initial, the system is
   A. numerical.
   B. alphabetical.
   C. color coded.
   D. limited.

_____ **7.** When files are organized in a variety of filing systems that place patient records one after the other in a pattern or an order, it is referred to as a
   A. tabbed order.
   B. labeled order.
   C. security order.
   D. sequential order.

_____ **8.** A new patient is
   A. always an infant.
   B. a patient who has never been seen in the practice before.
   C. a patient who has never been seen in the practice before or has not been seen in the practice in 3 years.
   D. never a patient who transferred from another practice.

_____ **9.** Another name for a reminder file is a(n)
   A. tickler file.
   B. supplemental file.
   C. retained file.
   D. inactive file.

_____ 10. Microfilm, microfiche, and cartridges
        A. require a lot of paper.
        B. are paperless.
        C. can be set up through a service.
        D. Both *B* and *C*

_____ 11. When selecting a commercial records center to assist with patient records, it is important to
        A. assess the monthly fee.
        B. assess the location.
        C. assess the system for retrieval and delivery of files.
        D. All of the above

_____ 12. Another name for hanging file folders is a(n)
        A. out guide.
        B. in guide.
        C. file jacket.
        D. file binder.

_____ 13. The proper order for the steps of filing is
        A. sort, inspect, code, index, and store.
        B. store, inspect, index, code, and sort.
        C. inspect, index, code, sort, and store.
        D. index, inspect, code, sort, and store.

_____ 14. The three categories of files are
        A. active, inactive, and closed.
        B. stored, deleted, and current.
        C. retained, returned, and indexed.
        D. locked, not locked, and highly confidential.

Sentence Completion

In the space provided, write the word or phrase that best completes each sentence.

_____ 15. Vertical files have a metal frame from which _____ are hung.

_____ 16. Whatever filing equipment is used, all files must be clearly _____ on the outside so they can be quickly located.

_____ 17. To protect the confidentiality of patient records, always keep them in a(n) _____ area.

_____ 18. _____ are large envelope-style folders with tabs in which files can be stored temporarily.

_____ 19. When there is a need to quickly identify files for categories of patients, such as Medicare patients, you might use a(n) _____ system.

_____ 20. If it becomes necessary to keep some patient information separate from the primary file, you might set up a(n) _____.

_____ 21. _____ is another term for naming a file.

_____ 22. When you put an identifying mark or phrase on a document to ensure that it is properly filed, you _____ it.

_____ **23.** The _____ must determine when a patient file should be considered inactive or closed.

_____ **24.** Use a(n) _____ to transfer paper files to a computer for storage.

Short Answer

Write the answer to each question on the lines provided.

25. Explain the advantage of compactible files over vertical or lateral files.

_____

_____

_____

26. Who should have keys to the file room? Why?

_____

_____

_____

27. What are two safety concerns when using filing equipment?

_____

_____

_____

28. What is the purpose of the tabs on file folders, and why are they positioned in different places on the folders?

_____

_____

_____

29. What is the purpose of the pockets on some out guides?

_____

_____

_____

30. What are two disadvantages of using a wall calendar as a tickler file?

_____

_____

_____

31. Name the five steps in the filing process.

_____

_____

_____

32. List six formats in which inactive and closed files can be stored.

_____

_____

_____

33. What security measures should an office manager take to ensure confidentiality when using a numeric system of filing?

_____

_____

_____

34. Describe a color coding system for patient filing. How might you set one up?

_____

_____

_____

35. Describe how supplemental files are different from primary medical records.

_____

_____

_____

36. Describe the "Inspecting" step in filing. What is included?

_____

_____

_____

37. Describe the steps to follow if a file is misplaced.

_____

_____

_____

Critical Thinking

Write the answer to each question on the lines provided.

1. Why is it important not to misplace patient files?

_____

_____

_____

2. How can the use of out guides help you locate misplaced files?

_____

_____

_____

3. What filing system would you choose for a practice that has many patients who are celebrities? Explain.

_____

_____

_____

4. How can color-coded patient files be helpful in the care and treatment of patients who have illnesses such as diabetes or HIV?

_____

_____

_____

5. What might be the consequences of destroying closed files too early?

_____

_____

_____

APPLICATIONS

Follow the directions for each application.

1. **Creating a Patient Filing System**

   Work in groups of four students. Within your group, choose partners to work together.

   a. With your partner, prepare a list of 15 hypothetical patients—complete with full names, ages, and primary ailments. Exchange patient lists with the other pair of students in your group.

   b. With your partner, analyze the patient list you have been given. Determine what kind of filing system, alphabetic or numeric, is appropriate.

   c. Organize the patients' names as you would for the filing system you have chosen. If you have chosen the alphabetic system, write each name on a different index card, and organize the cards. If you have chosen the numeric system, create a master list that shows the numbers and the corresponding patient names.

   d. Assume that your patient list is part of a much larger filing system that contains a similar mix of patients. Color-code your filing system. With your partner, decide what categories of information you need to identify through color coding. Then assign colors to your patient list as appropriate.

   e. After you have completed your filing system, meet with the other pair of students in your group and compare filing systems. How are they different? How are they alike? Each pair should evaluate the other pair's filing system for appropriateness and accuracy. Pairs should be able to justify their choices.

   f. Form different groups of four students. Exchange your original patient list with a different pair of students, and repeat steps **b** through **e**.

2. **Setting Up a Tickler File**

   Work with two partners. Two of you are medical assistants in charge of setting up a tickler file. The third partner is an evaluator.

   a. On the chalkboard, each student in the class should list one important date or activity that he needs to be reminded of weekly, monthly, or annually.

   b. Working together, the two medical assistants should analyze the reminder information to be included in the tickler file. Decide how you will organize the tickler file. Will you use file folders, a wall chart, a calendar, a binder, or a computer file? Create the tickler file.

c. Have the evaluator critique the tickler file. Her critique should answer these questions: Has any information been overlooked, misplaced, or duplicated? Is the tickler file accurate? Will it help in the day-to-day workings of an office?

d. As a group, discuss the evaluator's comments, noting the strengths and weaknesses of the tickler file as well as its accuracy and completeness.

e. Exchange roles and repeat the activity, choosing a different way of organizing the tickler file.

f. Exchange roles again so that each member of the group has an opportunity to set up and evaluate a tickler file.

CASE STUDIES

Write your response to each case study on the lines provided.

Case 1

You are in charge of the patient filing system for an office with four doctors. The system seems efficient, except that there is no way of knowing who has removed a particular file. You have had to go on numerous searches for missing files only to find them on someone's desk. What change could you make to the system to reduce the need to search the office for missing files?

_____

_____

_____

Case 2

You work for a large practice. The office manager and each doctor keep a separate tickler file. As a result, when one of these people is out sick or on vacation, important tasks are overlooked. What recommendations would you make for correcting this problem?

_____

_____

_____

Case 3

You have noticed that the patient files in your office contain medical records going back many years. It is becoming increasingly difficult to sort through all the documents and locate current medical information in a file. What can be done to solve this problem?

_____

_____

_____

Case 4

Your medical office has been storing inactive and closed paper files in a small storage space in the basement of the office building. That space is no longer adequate for all the files. The doctor has asked you to find space at an outside storage facility. What questions will you ask about a facility before selecting one?

_____

_____

_____

PROCEDURE COMPETENCY CHECKLISTS

PROCEDURE 10.1   Creating a Filing System for Patient Records

This procedure includes evaluating various filing systems and choosing the appropriate one. Steps for setting up the system and using it are also included.

Complete the steps below. A scoring system has been provided for each procedure. The total score for each individual procedure is 100 points. Each step within the procedure is weighted according to the importance of that step and is noted in the column "Point Value." Steps that are of a more critical nature have been weighted with a higher point value. Record your points for each step in the column "Points Achieved."

Determine your mastery of each step in the procedure by assigning it a score of 1 to 4 in the last column: 1 = poor, 2 = fair, 3 = good, 4 = excellent.

On the basis of your scores, budget time for additional practice of specific steps.

Materials: Vertical or horizontal filing cabinets with locks, file jackets, tabbed file folders, labels, file guides, out guides, filing sorters

Step	Point Value	Points Achieved	Mastery
1. Evaluate which filing system is best for your office—alphabetic or numeric. Make sure the doctor approves the system you choose.	20		
2. Establish a style for labeling files; use it for all labels. Place records for different family members in separate files.	15		
3. Set up a color-coding system to distinguish the files (for example, use blue for the letters A–C, red for D–F, and so on).	10		
4. Use file guides to divide files into sections.	10		
5. Use out guides to indicate which files have been removed. Include a charge-out form to be signed and dated by the person who is taking the file.	10		
6. To keep files in order and to avoid misplacing them, use a file sorter to hold records until they can be returned to the files.	15		
7. Develop a manual explaining the filing system to new staff members. Include guidelines on how to keep the system in good order.	10		
8. Avoid writing by hand. Type or use a label marker.	10		

Time limit: 10 minutes   Add Points Achieved: _____

Observer's Name: _____

Steps that require more practice: _____

_____

Instructor comments: _____

_____

_____

Name _____ Class _____ Date _____

PROCEDURE 10.2 Setting Up an Office Tickler File

This procedure outlines the steps for creating and utilizing a reminder file system.

Complete the steps below. A scoring system has been provided for each procedure. The total score for each individual procedure is 100 points. Each step within the procedure is weighted according to the importance of that step and is noted in the column "Point Value." Steps that are of a more critical nature have been weighted with a higher point value. Record your points for each step in the column "Points Achieved."

Determine your mastery of each step in the procedure by assigning it a score of 1 to 4 in the last column: 1 = poor, 2 = fair, 3 = good, 4 = excellent.

On the basis of your scores, budget time for additional practice of specific steps.

Materials: 12 manila file folders, 12 file labels, pen or typewriter, paper

Step	Point Value	Points Achieved	Mastery
1. Write or type 12 file labels, 1 for each month of the year. Abbreviations are acceptable. Do not include the year.	10		
2. Affix one label to the tab of each of 12 file folders.	10		
3. Arrange the folders so that the current month is on the top of the pile. Months should follow in chronological order.	10		
4. Make a list of upcoming responsibilities and activities and the date they should be completed. Use a separate sheet of paper for each month.	10		
5. File the notes by month in the appropriate folders.	10		
6. Place the folders, with the current month on top, in a prominent place in the office.	10		
7. Check the tickler file at least once a week on a specific day. Assign a backup person to check it if you are out of the office.	10		
8. Complete the tickler activities on the designated days. Keep notes concerning activities in progress. Discard old notes.	10		
9. At the end of the month, place that month's folder at the bottom of the tickler file. Move any remaining notes into the new month's folder.	10		
10. Continue to add new notes to the appropriate tickler files.	10		

Time limit: 10 minutes   Add Points Achieved: _____

Observer's Name: _____

Steps that require more practice: _____

Instructor comments: _____

PROCEDURE 10.3   Developing a Records Retention Program

This procedure includes identifying the types of information to be kept; researching the legal requirements of records retention; and developing, implementing, and periodically reviewing a system of records retention.

Complete the steps below. A scoring system has been provided for each procedure. The total score for each individual procedure is 100 points. Each step within the procedure is weighted according to the importance of that step and is noted in the column "Point Value." Steps that are of a more critical nature have been weighted with a higher point value. Record your points for each step in the column "Points Achieved."

Determine your mastery of each step in the procedure by assigning it a score of 1 to 4 in the last column: 1 = poor, 2 = fair, 3 = good, 4 = excellent.

On the basis of your scores, budget time for additional practice of specific steps.

Materials: *Guide to Record Retention Requirements* (published annually by the federal government), names and telephone numbers of local medical associations and state offices (including the state insurance commissioner and the medical practice's attorney), file folders, index cards, index box, paper, pen or typewriter

Step	Point Value	Points Achieved	Mastery
1. List the types of information in a typical patient medical record in your office. For example, a file for an adult patient may include the patient's case history, records of hospital stays, and insurance information.	5		
2. Research the legal, state, and federal requirements for keeping documents. Consult the *Guide to Record Retention Requirements* for federal guidelines. Contact the appropriate state office for specific state requirements. Call local medical associations. If your office does business in other states, research all applicable regulations. Consult with the attorney who represents your practice.	10		
3. Compile the results of your research in a chart. At the top of the chart, list the kinds of information your office keeps in patient records. Down the left side of the chart, list the headings Legal, Federal, State, and Other. In each box, record the corresponding information.	10		
4. Compare all the legal and government requirements. Indicate which one covers the longest period of time.	10		
5. Review the information with the doctor. Together, prepare a retention schedule. Decide how long different records should be kept in the office after a patient leaves the practice and how long records will be kept in storage. Because retention periods can vary for different types of information kept in a file, choose a retention period that covers all records. Determine how files will be destroyed when they have exceeded the retention period. Usually records are destroyed by paper shredding. Purchase any needed equipment.	5		

(continued)

Step	Point Value	Points Achieved	Mastery
6. Put the retention schedule in writing, post it prominently near the files, and review it with the staff. Keep a copy in a safe place.	5		
7. Develop a system for identifying files easily under the retention system. You might prepare an index card or create a master list for each inactive or closed file. It should include the patient's name and Social Security number, contents of the file, date the file was deemed inactive and by whom, date the file should be sent to storage (the actual date will be filled in later; if more than one storage location is used, indicate the location), date the file should be destroyed (the actual date will be filled in later). Have the card signed by the doctor and the person responsible for the files. Keep the card in an index box. This is your authorization to destroy the file at the appropriate time.	10		
8. Use color coding to help identify inactive files.	5		
9. One person should be responsible for checking the index cards each month to determine which files should be destroyed. Before retrieving files from storage, circulate a notice to the office staff stating which records will be destroyed. Indicate that they must let you know by a specific date if any files should be saved. You may keep a separate file with these notices.	10		
10. After the deadline has passed, retrieve the files from storage. Review each file. Make sure staff members who will be destroying the files are trained to use the equipment. Develop an instruction sheet describing how to destroy files. Post it prominently with the retention schedule and near the machinery used to destroy the files.	10		
11. Update the index card, giving the date the file was destroyed and by whom.	10		
12. Periodically review the retention schedule. Update it with current legal and governmental requirements. With the staff, evaluate whether the current schedule is meeting the needs of your office or whether files are being kept too long or destroyed prematurely. With the doctor's approval, change the schedule as necessary.	10		

Time limit: 10 minutes   Add Points Achieved: _____

Observer's Name: _____

Steps that require more practice: _____

_____

Instructor comments: _____

_____

_____

CHAPTER 11

Telephone Techniques

REVIEW

Vocabulary Review

Matching

Match the key terms in the right column with the definitions in the left column by placing the letter of each correct answer in the space provided.

_____ 1. telephone etiquette

_____ 2. tone

_____ 3. pronunciation

_____ 4. enunciation

_____ 5. pitch

_____ 6. routing list

_____ 7. telephone answering system

_____ 8. facsimile machine

_____ 9. ARU telephone system

_____ 10. triage

a. speaking in a positive, respectful manner
b. good manners
c. fax machine
d. telecommunication
e. screening and sorting of emergency incidents
f. high or low level of speech
g. specifies who is responsible for various types of calls and how the calls are to be handled
h. automated voicemail system
i. saying words correctly
j. clear and distinct speaking

Passage Completion

Study the key terms in the box. Use your textbook to find definitions of terms you do not understand.

| enunciation | pitch | telephone triage |
| etiquette | pronunciation | |

In the space provided, complete the following passage, using the terms from the box. You may change the form of a term to fit the meaning of the sentence.

The telephone is an important tool in today's medical practice. How you handle telephone calls will have an impact on the public image of the office. When speaking on the telephone, always use proper telephone (11) _____ to present a positive impression of the office. Make your voice pleasant and effective by varying your (12) _____. Remember not to mumble. Good (13) _____ will help the caller understand the important information you are trying to convey. Proper (14) _____ of the caller's name will help her feel welcome and important. In today's medical practice, the process of determining the level of urgency of each call and how it should be handled or routed is called (15) _____.

11. _____

12. _____

13. _____

14. _____

15. _____

Content Review

Multiple Choice

In the space provided, write the letter of the choice that best completes each statement or answers each question.

_____ 1. The first thing you should do when answering a call is
   A. schedule an appointment for the caller.
   B. put the caller on hold.
   C. find out who is calling.
   D. alert the doctor that a patient is calling.

_____ 2. Which of the following types of calls would a medical assistant handle?
   A. A call to cancel an appointment
   B. A call to discuss abnormal test results
   C. An emergency call
   D. A call from another doctor

_____ 3. If a caller refuses to discuss his symptoms with anyone but the physician,
   A. schedule an appointment immediately.
   B. route the call to another medical assistant.
   C. have the doctor return the call.
   D. call the patient the next day to see whether he has changed his mind.

_____ 4. After speaking with a patient on the telephone, a medical assistant must always
   A. meet with the doctor to discuss the call.
   B. schedule an appointment for the patient.
   C. bill the patient for the telephone time.
   D. document the conversation.

_____ 5. When a patient has difficulty paying a bill, it is usually acceptable for the
   A. doctor to stop treatment.
   B. patient to switch to another doctor.
   C. doctor to stop scheduling appointments.
   D. patient to pay the bill in installments.

_____ 6. It is not a good idea for a patient to use old medication because
  A. the patient will have difficulty getting the prescription renewed.
  B. the medication may no longer be effective.
  C. the patient may not have enough of the old medication.
  D. only extreme illnesses require any medication at all.

_____ 7. If a caller asks for medical advice from a medical assistant, the assistant should
  A. hang up immediately.
  B. offer advice but stress that it is only her opinion.
  C. refuse to give advice and urge the patient to see the physician.
  D. insist that the caller go to the nearest emergency room.

_____ 8. Emergency calls must be
  A. immediately routed to the physician.
  B. put on hold while the assistant calls 911.
  C. routed to a nurse practitioner.
  D. considered pranks until proven otherwise.

_____ 9. A medical assistant may release patient information to an outside caller
  A. only when that caller is an attorney.
  B. only when that caller is a physician.
  C. only when requested to do so by the physician.
  D. whenever it is requested.

_____ 10. After you have taken a message from a caller,
  A. leave the message on your desk.
  B. repeat the key points to the caller for verification.
  C. put the caller on hold.
  D. mark the message confidential and file it.

_____ 11. The most common calls to a medical office are
  A. administrative.
  B. clinical.
  C. emergencies.
  D. solicitation.

_____ 12. Which of the following types of telephone calls can a medical assistant handle?
  A. Reports from patients concerning unsatisfactory progress
  B. A patient requesting x-ray results
  C. A call to change an appointment
  D. A call from another doctor

_____ 13. If you are uncertain about giving particular information to a patient, a general principle is to
  A. have the nurse relay the information.
  B. document the details of the call, including what you said, in the chart.
  C. realize that it is appropriate and honest to give information to the patient.
  D. have the physician return the patient's call.

_____ 14. If a patient remains dissatisfied after discussing a bill,
  A. document all comments and relay the information to the physician.
  B. tell the patient that you are sorry he is dissatisfied, but the bill stands as is.
  C. turn the patient's bill over to a collection agency.
  D. terminate the patient's care until the bill is paid.

_____ 15. When may a medical assistant authorize a pharmacy to refill a prescription?
      A. Never
      B. If it is a regular medication for the patient
      C. If the physician has authorized on the patient's chart that refills are approved
      D. Only if the medical assistant has knowledge of the medication

Sentence Completion

In the space provided, write the word or phrase that best completes each sentence.

_____ 16. The medical assistant handles calls that deal with _____ issues.

_____ 17. A(n) _____ specifies who is responsible for the various types of calls in the office and how the calls are to be handled.

_____ 18. If you will be discussing clinical matters over the telephone, it is a good idea to pull the _____.

_____ 19. A medical assistant may authorize a pharmacy to renew a prescription only when the physician _____ in the patient's chart.

_____ 20. The medical assistant may be responsible for making routine _____ to verify that patients are following treatment instructions.

_____ 21. Before putting a call on hold, ask the caller to state the reason for the call so that you do not inadvertently put a(n) _____ on hold.

_____ 22. When giving information over the telephone, always ask whether the caller has any _____ about what you have discussed.

_____ 23. It is always a good idea to complete a call by _____ the important points of the conversation and thanking the caller.

_____ 24. When taking a telephone message, always record the date and _____ of the call.

_____ 25. The medical assistant must maintain patient _____ when handling written telephone messages.

Short Answer

Write the answer to each question on the lines provided.

26. List seven symptoms or conditions that would qualify as medical emergencies.

_____

_____

_____

27. List three types of calls that a medical assistant would handle.

_____

_____

_____

28. List the five Cs of communication, and explain what each means.

_____

_____

_____

29. List seven types of incoming calls that a medical assistant can handle.

_____

_____

_____

30. List at least ten symptoms or conditions that would qualify as a medical emergency.

_____

_____

_____

31. What are five ways you can make your telephone voice effective?

_____

_____

_____

32. What is the typical procedure for putting a call on hold?

_____

_____

_____

33. How is telephone triage conducted?

_____

_____

_____

_____

Critical Thinking

Write the answer to each question on the lines provided.

1. How can the telephone image you present have an impact on public perception of your medical office?

_____

_____

_____

2. Compare and contrast the way you would respond to a caller inquiring about a bill and a caller requesting the results of laboratory tests.

_____

_____

_____

3. Describe how a medical assistant might respond when a patient calls the office to discuss symptoms she is experiencing.

_____

_____

_____

4. If a patient calls with an emergency situation and can only stay on the telephone for 1 minute, what questions would be the most important to ask?

_____

_____

_____

5. How does a well-trained, efficient telephone staff benefit the physician?

_____

_____

_____

6. Discuss how you would respond to a patient who calls to inquire about his abnormal lab results.

_____

_____

_____

7. Discuss how you would respond to a patient who calls to request a prescription refill.

_____

_____

_____

8. Describe what triage is.

_____

_____

_____

APPLICATIONS

Follow the directions for each application.

1. **Handling a Patient Call**

   Work with two partners. Have one partner play the role of an angry patient calling to complain about being billed for a procedure that never took place. Have the second partner act as a medical assistant handling the call. Have the third partner act as an observer and evaluator.

   a. Role-play the telephone call. The medical assistant should listen carefully to the caller, taking notes about the details of the problem. The medical assistant should also be sure to ask all necessary questions.

   b. The medical assistant should respond to the caller's complaint in a professional manner and explain the specific action that will be taken to address the issue.

   c. Have the observer provide a critique of the medical assistant's handling of the call. The critique should evaluate the use of proper telephone etiquette, the proper routing of the call, and the assistant's telephone notes. Comments should include both positive feedback and suggestions for improvement.

   d. Exchange roles and repeat the exercise. Allow the student playing the caller to choose another reason for the call.

   e. Exchange roles again so that each member of the group has an opportunity to play the role of the medical assistant.

   f. Discuss the strengths and weaknesses of each group member's telephone etiquette.

2. **Taking Telephone Messages**

   Work with a partner to design the best possible telephone message pad or telephone log for a medical office.

   a. Consider the various types of incoming calls that the medical practice receives. Review the different types of information that a person taking a message might need to obtain. Make a list of the types of calls and types of information. Think about the order in which the information is obtained. Decide how much space is needed for each entry.

   b. Choose which you will design—a telephone message pad or telephone log. As you work with your partner to design it, consider these questions: What is the best size for the pad or log? How many messages will fit on one page? How will copies be made? What color will the pad or log be? Pay attention to the information that must be included, the space available for each message, and the layout of the page.

   c. Test your telephone message pad or log. Have your partner role-play a patient calling a medical office. Use your message pad or log to take the message.

   d. Then trade roles and repeat the role playing. Discuss the strengths and weaknesses of your message pad or log. Revise your design as needed.

   e. Share your message pad or log with other pairs of students. Critique each other's designs. Discuss how the designs are different and how they are similar. Assess the strengths and weaknesses of each design. Offer suggestions for revisions.

   f. Make final adjustments to the design of your telephone message pad or telephone log on the basis of your classmates' feedback.

Name _____ Class _____ Date _____

CASE STUDIES

Write your response to each case study on the lines provided.

Case 1

A patient calls and demands to speak with the doctor but refuses to identify herself. What should you do?

_____

_____

_____

Case 2

Mr. Suzuki calls the medical office to schedule an appointment and to request a prescription renewal. What can you, the medical assistant, handle?

_____

_____

_____

Case 3

In one morning, you receive calls from a patient with an emergency, an attorney, a physician from another medical office, and a salesperson. Describe how you would route each of these calls.

_____

_____

_____

Case 4

You observe a coworker taking a telephone call. After answering the call by giving her name and the office name, she listens quietly. She then asks how to pronounce the caller's name. A few minutes later she slams down the receiver. She immediately storms off to lunch. What did your coworker do correctly? What did she do incorrectly? Explain.

_____

_____

_____

Case 5

Mrs. Rosetti calls the office and discusses a confidential medical problem with you. How should you handle this situation?

_____

_____

_____

Case 6

The doctor asks you to arrange a patient consultation with another physician in the area. Outline the procedure you would follow.

_____

_____

_____

PROCEDURE COMPETENCY CHECKLISTS

PROCEDURE 11.1   Handling Emergency Calls

This procedure outlines the appropriate steps to be taken during an emergency call, including obtaining necessary information and responding appropriately.

Complete the steps below. A scoring system has been provided for each procedure. The total score for each individual procedure is 100 points. Each step within the procedure is weighted according to the importance of that step and is noted in the column "Point Value." Steps that are of a more critical nature have been weighted with a higher point value. Record your points for each step in the column "Points Achieved."

Determine your mastery of each step in the procedure by assigning it a score of 1 to 4 in the last column: 1 = poor, 2 = fair, 3 = good, 4 = excellent.

On the basis of your scores, budget time for additional practice of specific steps.

Materials: Office guidelines for handling emergency calls; list of symptoms and conditions requiring immediate medical attention; telephone numbers of area emergency rooms, poison control centers, and ambulance transport services; telephone message pads or telephone message log

Step	Point Value	Points Achieved	Mastery
1. When someone calls the office regarding a potential emergency, remain calm.	20		

2. Obtain the following information:
  a. The caller's name
  b. The caller's relation to the patient
  c. The patient's name
  d. The patient's age
  e. A description of the patient's symptoms
  f. A description of how the accident or injury occurred
  g. A description of the patient's reaction to the situation
  h. Any treatment that has been administered
  i. The caller's telephone number and the address from which the call is being made
	20		

3. Read back the details of the medical problem to verify them.	15		
4. If necessary, refer to the list of symptoms and conditions that require immediate medical attention to determine whether the situation is an emergency.	10		

5. **If the situation is a medical emergency,** put the call through to the doctor immediately. If the doctor is not in the office, follow established office procedures. They may involve:
  a. Transferring the call to the nurse practitioner or other medical personnel
  b. Instructing the caller to dial 911 to request an ambulance
  c. Instructing the patient to go to the nearest emergency room
  d. Instructing the caller to telephone the nearest poison control center for advice and supplying the telephone number
  e. Paging the doctor
	15		

(continued)

Step	Point Value	Points Achieved	Mastery
6. **If the situation is not a medical emergency,** handle the call according to established office procedures.	10		
7. If you are in doubt about whether the situation is an emergency, treat it as an emergency.	10		

Time limit: 10 minutes   Add Points Achieved: _____

Observer's Name: _____

Steps that require more practice: _____
_____

Instructor comments: _____
_____
_____

PROCEDURE 11.2   Retrieving Messages From an Answering Service

This procedure includes setting a schedule for and gathering the appropriate information from the routing of retrieved messages.

Complete the steps below. A scoring system has been provided for each procedure. The total score for each individual procedure is 100 points. Each step within the procedure is weighted according to the importance of that step and is noted in the column "Point Value." Steps that are of a more critical nature have been weighted with a higher point value. Record your points for each step in the column "Points Achieved."

Determine your mastery of each step in the procedure by assigning it a score of 1 to 4 in the last column: 1 = poor, 2 = fair, 3 = good, 4 = excellent.

On the basis of your scores, budget time for additional practice of specific steps.

Materials: Telephone message pad or telephone log

Step	Point Value	Points Achieved	Mastery
1. Set a regular schedule for calling the answering service to retrieve messages.	15		
2. Call at the regularly scheduled time(s) to see whether there are any messages.	15		
3. Identify yourself, and state that you are calling to obtain messages for the practice.	15		
4. Write down all pertinent information for each message on the telephone message pad or telephone log. Be sure to include the patient's name and telephone number, time of call, message or description of the problem, and any action taken.	25		

(continued)

Step	Point Value	Points Achieved	Mastery
5. Repeat the information, confirming that you have the correct spelling of all names.	15		
6. When you have retrieved all messages, route them according to the office policy.	15		

Time limit: 10 minutes

Add Points Achieved: _____

Observer's Name: _____

Steps that require more practice: _____

_____

Instructor comments: _____

_____

_____

CHAPTER **12**

Scheduling Appointments and Maintaining the Physician's Schedule

REVIEW

Vocabulary Review

Matching

Match the key terms in the right column with the definitions in the left column by placing the letter of each correct answer in the space provided.

_____ 1. A scheduling system in which patients arrive at their own convenience, knowing that they will be seen on a first-come, first-served basis

_____ 2. A scheduling system in which patients are scheduled at regular, specific times throughout the day

_____ 3. A scheduling system in which several patients are given the same appointment time but are taken as they arrive so that the office schedule remains on track each hour even if patients are late

_____ 4. An adaptation of the system described in no. 3, in which patients might be scheduled in certain increments, allowing time to catch up before the next hour begins

_____ 5. A scheduling system in which two or more patients are scheduled for the same appointment slot, with the expectation that both patients will be seen by the doctor within the scheduled period

_____ 6. A scheduling system in which similar appointments are grouped together during the day or week

_____ 7. A scheduling system in which patients are booked weeks or months ahead of time

_____ 8. A patient who arrives without an appointment and still expects to see the doctor

_____ 9. A patient who does not come to his appointment

_____ 10. Scheduling more patients than reasonably can be expected to be seen in the time allowed

_____ 11. Leaving large, unused gaps in the schedule

_____ 12. A detailed travel plan that lists dates and times of flights and events, locations of meetings and lodgings, and relevant telephone numbers

a. time-specified scheduling
b. overbooking
c. minutes
d. open-hours scheduling
e. itinerary
f. walk-in
g. wave scheduling
h. advance scheduling
i. modified-wave scheduling
j. double-booking system
k. cluster scheduling
l. no-show
m. agenda
n. locum tenens
o. underbooking

_____ **13.** A substitute physician

_____ **14.** A list of topics to be discussed or presented at a meeting

_____ **15.** A report of what was discussed and decided at a meeting

Content Review

Multiple Choice

In the space provided, write the letter of the choice that best completes each statement or answers each question.

_____ **1.** A system used typically in emergency centers rather than in private practice is
   A. modified-wave scheduling.
   B. double booking.
   C. open-hours scheduling.
   D. cluster scheduling.

_____ **2.** What is the purpose of a recall notice?
   A. It reminds a patient that the time has come to make an appointment that was too far away from her last appointment for the booking system to accommodate.
   B. It alerts the patient to a change in the physician's plans (for example, attendance at a medical conference) and asks the patient to call the office to reschedule the appointment.
   C. It is used when a reminder mailing fails to reach the patient.
   D. It notifies a patient from a referring physician that the patient's appointment for a second opinion has been scheduled.

_____ **3.** If a patient comes in unexpectedly with an emergency condition, it is vital that
   A. the nearest hospital be notified immediately.
   B. the patient be treated as quickly as the schedule will allow.
   C. a physician see that patient ahead of patients who may already be waiting.
   D. patients who have appointments at that time be given the chance to reschedule.

_____ **4.** A disadvantage of the wave scheduling system is that
   A. patients may have a considerable wait before seeing the physician.
   B. patients become annoyed or angry when realizing they have appointments at the same time as other patients.
   C. it prevents the medical assistant from pulling the patients' charts before they arrive.
   D. it assume that two patients will actually be seen by the doctor within the scheduled period.

_____ **5.** What type of appointment scheduling system can be helpful if a patient calls and needs to be seen that day but no appointments are available?
   A. Double-booking
   B. Wave
   C. Modified-wave
   D. Cluster

_____ **6.** Which appointment scheduling system determines the number of patients to be seen each hour by dividing the hour by the length of the average visit?
   A. Double-booking
   B. Cluster
   C. Wave
   D. Advance

_____ 7. The appropriate procedure to follow for a patient who misses an appointment is to
   A. document the no-show in the appointment book and in the patient's chart.
   B. notify the patient that she will be charged for the missed appointment and interest will be applied.
   C. refuse to reschedule an appointment for the patient.
   D. schedule another appointment for the patient but tell her she must call the day before or the appointment will be canceled.

_____ 8. What should you do when a pharmaceutical sales representative that you do not know comes to the office without an appointment?
   A. Tell him to have a seat and notify the physician.
   B. Ask him to leave a business card.
   C. Take him directly to see the physician.
   D. Have him give you all the information.

_____ 9. Obtaining patient information for an appointment should include which of the following?
   A. Marital status
   B. Religion
   C. Purpose of the visit
   D. Occupation

_____ 10. Before scheduling an outside appointment for a patient, the medical assistant must
   A. obtain an order from the doctor for the exact procedure to be performed.
   B. talk with the patient to find convenient appointment times.
   C. ask the patient if she would rather schedule the appointment.
   D. determine the day and time the procedure must be performed.

_____ 11. What does the abbreviation CP stand for?
   A. Canceled procedure
   B. Complains politely
   C. Check progress
   D. Chest pain

_____ 12. Most minor medical problems, such as a sore throat, earache, or blood sugar check, usually require how many minutes?
   A. 10 to 15
   B. 15 to 20
   C. 20 to 30
   D. 30 to 45

_____ 13. The abbreviation Rx stands for?
   A. X-ray procedure
   B. Treatment
   C. Prescription
   D. Immunization

_____ 14. The correct abbreviation for blood pressure is
   A. Bld P.
   B. BP.
   C. BPr.
   D. BLPr.

_____ 15. Appointments that are anticipated to require more time should be scheduled
    A. at the beginning of the hour.
    B. at the end of the hour.
    C. with another patient's 10-minute time slot.
    D. during a 10-minute time slot.

_____ 16. The appointment book is a legal record and should be kept at least
    A. 1 year.
    B. 6 months.
    C. 3 years.
    D. 1 month.

Sentence Completion

In the space provided, write the word or phrase that best completes each sentence.

_____ 17. The first step in preparing the appointment book is to determine the _____, or basic format.

_____ 18. To save time when entering information in the appointment book, you could use the standard abbreviation CPE to stand for _____.

_____ 19. Various types of _____ include open-hours, time-specified, wave, modified-wave, double-booking, cluster, advance, and combination.

_____ 20. _____ scheduling systems can be programmed to lock out selected appointment slots, which can be saved for emergencies.

_____ 21. Filling out a(n) _____ and handing it to the patient helps remind the patient about an upcoming appointment.

_____ 22. To see a referral on relatively short notice is a matter of _____ to the referring physician.

_____ 23. If empty spaces are created in the schedule because patients have called to _____, you may be able to arrange to have other patients come in earlier than planned.

_____ 24. Appointments are often made outside the medical office for surgeries, consultations with other physicians, and various _____ tests.

_____ 25. Taking careful _____ makes it relatively easy to report on the meeting of a professional society or committee.

_____ 26. Making travel arrangements for a physician may include securing airline reservations, requesting _____ of room reservations, and picking up tickets.

Short Answer

Write the answer to each question on the lines provided.

27. After arriving at the office, about how long is the average patient willing to wait to see a physician? Why?

_____

_____

_____

28. How can having a list of standard procedures and the time required for each procedure help you be an efficient scheduler?

_____

_____

_____

29. What main factors determine the type of appointment scheduling system a medical office uses?

_____

_____

_____

30. How does time-specified scheduling work?

_____

_____

_____

31. Name three factors that would determine the need for reminder calls.

_____

_____

_____

32. Give three examples of special scheduling situations that would require you to adjust the schedule for patient needs.

_____

_____

_____

33. What special needs should you consider when booking a patient with diabetes?

_____

_____

_____

34. Why is it beneficial to involve the patient in scheduling his outside appointments?

_____

_____

_____

35. If a pharmaceutical sales representative requests an appointment with the doctor, how should you proceed?

_____

_____

_____

36. What is an agenda?

_____

_____

_____

37. What are the minutes of a meeting?

_____

_____

_____

38. Define locum tenens.

_____

_____

_____

39. What does the abbreviation c/o stand for?

_____

_____

_____

40. What does the abbreviation GI stand for?

_____

_____

_____

Critical Thinking

Write the answer to each question on the lines provided.

1. What are two things you could learn from patients who are chronically late for appointments?

_____

_____

_____

2. Why might physicians prefer to schedule new patients first thing in the morning?

_____

_____

_____

3. Why might underbooking be a cause of stress within a medical office?

_____

_____

_____

4. What types of practices may require more than one locum tenens on call to cover during a physician's absence?

_____

_____

_____

5. Why is it preferable for you, not the patient, to take the responsibility for scheduling patient appointments outside the office?

_____

_____

_____

6. Why is it important to document no-shows or canceled appointments in a patient's chart?

_____

_____

_____

7. Name three factors that would determine the need for reminder calls.

_____

_____

_____

8. List the information you need to book a patient's appointment.

_____

_____

_____

9. Describe the proper way to document a cancellation or a no-show in the appointment book.

_____

_____

_____

APPLICATIONS

Follow the directions for each application.

1. Scheduling Appointments

Schedule your classmates for appointments at a medical practice.

a. Choose the type of specialty for the practice and the days and hours that the office will be open to see patients each week. Select a scheduling system for your office to use.

b. Determine five procedures (checkups, minor in-office surgeries, and so on) to be performed at the practice. Estimate the typical length of time for each procedure.

c. Schedule the students in your class for appointments, making sure that there is enough time for the procedures to be performed. For each appointment, record the patient's full name, home and work telephone numbers, purpose of visit, and estimated length of visit. Use abbreviations where helpful.

d. Evaluate the schedule for overbooking or underbooking. Share your schedule with another student and ask for comments. Revise the schedule as necessary.

2. **Developing a Travel Itinerary**

A physician in your practice is attending the American Medical Association's annual conference, to be held at the Hyatt Regency Hotel in Chicago. Develop a travel itinerary that you can give to the physician and also keep a copy of in the office for reference.

a. Determine the dates of the conference and the dates of the physician's departure and return. Choose the airline that the physician will fly, and note the flight times.

b. Record the itinerary in chronological order. Include telephone numbers and addresses of each location where the physician can be reached as well as the dates and times that the physician can be reached there.

c. Evaluate your itinerary. Are you able to contact the physician at every point during the trip? If not, is there additional information you can list on the itinerary?

d. Examine itineraries developed by your classmates. Is there something they included in their itineraries that you can add to yours?

e. With your classmates, discuss the value of having an itinerary.

CASE STUDIES

Write your response to each case study on the lines provided.

Case 1

When you check the appointment book for today's schedule, you realize the page is missing. What steps can you take to resolve the situation?

_____

_____

_____

Case 2

A female patient becomes upset when a man who just arrived at the office is taken to see the doctor immediately. The woman has been waiting for almost an hour and was supposed to be seen next. What should you do?

_____

_____

_____

Case 3

A medical assistant informs waiting patients that the physician will be delayed. She shares details about the emergency appendectomy the mayor's daughter needs, which will take at least an hour. She asks patients whether they prefer to wait, reschedule, or run errands and come back later. Has the medical assistant handled this situation appropriately? Explain.

_____

_____

_____

_____

Case 4

Many patients have complained about the long wait at the medical office in which you work. The office manager asks you to develop a system to track the time it takes patients to complete their visits. Describe the system that you would develop.

_____

_____

_____

PROCEDURE COMPETENCY CHECKLISTS

PROCEDURE 12.1   Creating a Cluster Schedule

This procedure includes establishing the types of cases to be clustered, determining the average length of a visit, and appropriately blocking off times in the schedule.

Complete the steps below. A scoring system has been provided for each procedure. The total score for each individual procedure is 100 points. Each step within the procedure is weighted according to the importance of that step and is noted in the column "Point Value." Steps that are of a more critical nature have been weighted with a higher point value. Record your points for each step in the column "Points Achieved."

Determine your mastery of each step in the procedure by assigning it a score of 1 to 4 in the last column: 1 = poor, 2 = fair, 3 = good, 4 = excellent.

On the basis of your scores, budget time for additional practice of specific steps.

Materials: Calendar, tickler file, appointment book, colored pencils or markers (optional)

Step	Point Value	Points Achieved	Mastery
1. Learn which categories of cases the physician would like to cluster and on what days and/or times of day.	20		
2. Determine the length of the average visit in each category.	20		
3. In the appointment book, cross out the hours in the week when the physician is typically not available.	20		
4. Block out one period in midmorning and one in midafternoon for use as buffer, or reserve, times for unexpected needs.	20		
5. Reserve additional slots for acutely ill patients.	10		
6. Mark the appointment times for clustered procedures. If desired, color-code the blocks of time.	10		

Time limit: 10 minutes   Add Points Achieved: _____

Observer's Name: _____

Steps that require more practice: _____

_____

Instructor comments: _____

_____

_____

PROCEDURE 12.2   Scheduling and Confirming Surgery at a Hospital

This procedure includes determining the urgency of the surgery, scheduling the procedure, arranging for admissions, providing preadmission forms, and confirming the scheduled appointment.

Complete the steps below. A scoring system has been provided for each procedure. The total score for each individual procedure is 100 points. Each step within the procedure is weighted according to the importance of that step and is noted in the column "Point Value." Steps that are of a more critical nature have been weighted with a higher point value. Record your points for each step in the column "Points Achieved."

Determine your mastery of each step in the procedure by assigning it a score of 1 to 4 in the last column: 1 = poor, 2 = fair, 3 = good, 4 = excellent.

On the basis of your scores, budget time for additional practice of specific steps.

Materials: Calendar, telephone, notepad, pen

Step	Point Value	Points Achieved	Mastery
1. Determine whether the need is for elective surgery or emergency surgery. Patients facing elective surgery may be given only one or two choices of days and times. For emergency surgery, the first step is to reserve the operating room.	25		
2. Call the operating room secretary. Give the procedure required, the name of the surgeon, the length of time involved, and the preferred date and hour.	15		
3. Provide the patient's name, address, telephone number, age, gender, Social Security number, and insurance information.	15		
4. Arrange with the admissions office for the patient to be admitted on the day of surgery or the day before (depending on the type of surgery). Ask for a copy of the admissions form for the patient record.	15		
5. If the hospital requires patients to complete preadmission forms, request a blank form for the patient.	15		
6. Confirm the surgery and the patient's arrival time 1 business day before surgery.	15		

Time limit: 10 minutes   Add Points Achieved: _____

Observer's Name: _____

Steps that require more practice: _____

_____

Instructor comments: _____

_____

_____

CHAPTER 13

Patient Reception Area

REVIEW

Vocabulary Review

True or False

Decide whether each statement is true or false. In the space at the left, write T for true or F for false. On the lines provided, rewrite the false statements to make them true.

_____ 1. An interim room allows patients some privacy while they talk with office staff.

_____

_____ 2. A bandage from a child's cut is infectious waste, but a used diaper is not.

_____

_____ 3. The Americans With Disabilities Act protects people against discrimination because of their age.

_____

_____ 4. A contagious disease can be spread among patients waiting in a reception area.

_____

_____ 5. People from different economic levels are considered to be differently abled.

_____

_____ 6. A color family is a group of colors that work well together.

_____

_____ 7. A two-story office building that does not have elevator service could be said to have good access.

_____

_____ 8. Patients should have clear, easy access from the parking lot to the medical office door.

_____

_____ 9. The Americans With Disabilities Act requires that doorways have a minimum width of 28 inches.

_____

_____ 10. A bulletin board is not appropriate in a medical practice.

_____

_____ **11.** Health magazines geared toward the general public are a good choice for reading material in a medical office.

_____

_____ **12.** The Older Americans Act of 1965 was passed by Congress to eliminate discrimination against the elderly.

_____

_____ **13.** Infectious waste is never cleaned up by a medical assistant.

_____

_____ **14.** No matter how tastefully it is decorated, the reception area will be unappealing if it is not clean.

_____

_____ **15.** The primary pastime in the patient reception areas is watching television.

_____

_____ **16.** Toys designed for outside use are appropriate for pediatric reception areas.

_____

Content Review

Multiple Choice

In the space provided, write the letter of the choice that best answers each question or completes each statement.

_____ **1.** Which of the following color combinations is considered harmonious?
   A. Red, orange, blue
   B. White, blue, mauve
   C. Red, hot pink, white
   D. Blue, mauve, yellow

_____ **2.** OSHA is a federal agency that
   A. oversees health practices.
   B. regulates citizens' health and safety.
   C. sets safety standards for the workplace.
   D. provides assistance to people with disabilities.

_____ **3.** A double door leading from the medical office to the outside of the building
   A. helps patients feel safe in the waiting area.
   B. discourages salespeople from entering.
   C. helps patients locate the office.
   D. minimizes drafts in the reception area.

_____ **4.** Which of the following items would be a good addition to a pediatrician's reception area?
   A. Videocassette recorder (VCR) and children's videotapes
   B. Sponge ball and bat
   C. Bag of marbles
   D. Bottle of bubble-blowing liquid

_____ 5. If the medical practice includes older people, choose reception room furniture that
  A. is soft and comfortable.
  B. includes some straight-backed chairs.
  C. is low to the floor to reduce falls.
  D. has no arms to get in the way.

_____ 6. The decor of the reception room
  A. doesn't matter because only the medical care is important.
  B. can create whatever impression is desired.
  C. is effective only if completed by a trained interior decorator.
  D. does not include carpeting.

_____ 7. The correct amount of furniture in a reception area
  A. is enough furniture so that all patients and family members or friends who accompany the patient can sit comfortably, no matter how busy the office schedule is.
  B. is 6 chairs and 1 sofa.
  C. is 10 chairs and no sofas.
  D. depends on the size of the room and the number of windows and is usually 6 to 8 chairs.

_____ 8. The interim room in a medical office is
  A. a room where a patient changes to a medical gown.
  B. the same as an examination room.
  C. where the medical equipment is stored.
  D. a room where people can talk or meet without being seen or heard from the patient reception area.

_____ 9. Pediatric reception areas are
  A. designed to meet the special size and needs of children.
  B. required under federal law for all family practice offices.
  C. different from traditional reception areas only in that all the furniture is smaller.
  D. designed only for sick children.

_____ 10. A cleaning communications notebook is
  A. a means of communication between the office staff and the cleaning staff.
  B. a way to list special cleanup needs for the cleaning staff.
  C. a way to congratulate and thank the cleaning staff.
  D. All of the above

_____ 11. A Telecom Teletype Machine
  A. is required by federal law in medical practices.
  B. looks just like a regular telephone.
  C. looks like a laptop computer with a cradle for the receiver of a traditional telephone.
  D. is not capable of communicating with another Telecom Teletype Machine.

_____ 12. The purpose of OSHA is
  A. to eliminate discrimination against the elderly.
  B. to eliminate discrimination against the disabled.
  C. to mandate federal safety precautions for the workplace.
  D. None of the above

Sentence Completion

In the space provided, write the word or phrase that best completes each sentence.

_____ 13. Older patients waiting in a reception area may feel colder than younger people because they have a(n) _____ metabolism.

_____ 14. Music in the reception area should reflect the interests of the _____.

_____ 15. Choose _____ plants for the reception area.

_____ 16. To make sure waiting patients do not feel crowded, allow _____ square feet of space per person.

_____ 17. In a large medical office, the cleaning service is often supervised by a(n) _____.

_____ 18. When removing stains from reception room furniture, use _____ water because it is unlikely to set the stains.

_____ 19. OSHA requires the regular use of _____ as part of a cleaning schedule.

_____ 20. To protect patients and staff from being trapped by a fire, medical offices are legally required to install _____.

_____ 21. To inform patients about area meetings, classes, support groups, health fairs, and speakers relating to the physician's specialty, you might set up a(n) _____ in the reception area.

_____ 22. To protect all patients, but especially those who are immuno-compromised, it is best to take _____ patients directly into the examination room.

Short Answer

Write the answer to each question on the lines provided.

23. How does the American Medical Association suggest calculating the amount of seating that should be in a physician's reception area?

_____

_____

_____

24. What are five daily tasks involved in cleaning a reception area?

_____

_____

_____

25. Why should you take special care in cleaning up after a patient who has vomited or bled on the furniture in the reception area?

_____

_____

_____

26. What are three factors to consider in determining the number of parking spaces a medical office needs?

_____

_____

_____

27. Why does the Americans With Disabilities Act require a minimum width for hallways?

_____

_____

_____

28. Give two reasons why a medical office should have at least two exits.

_____

_____

_____

29. What are four types of appropriate reading material for the patient reception area?

_____

_____

_____

30. Why should all medical offices, not just those visited by patients in wheelchairs, provide ramps?

_____

_____

_____

31. List three ways you could make a reception area more comfortable for elderly patients.

_____

_____

_____

32. List four aspects of a reception area that can make a stay there seem longer than it actually is.

_____

_____

_____

33. List five steps for cleaning stains.

_____

_____

_____

34. List six guidelines for safety in the reception area.

_____

_____

_____

35. List three cool colors.

_____

_____

_____

36. List three warm colors.

_____

_____

_____

37. List five items that may appropriately be found on a medical office bulletin board.

_____

_____

_____

Critical Thinking

Write the answer to each question on the lines provided.

1. Why would big-band music or classical music be a poor choice for background music in a pediatric practice? What type of music would be better?

_____

_____

_____

2. If patients are happy with their doctor, what difference does it make if the furniture and decor of the reception area are out of date or a little worn?

_____

_____

_____

3. What kind of specialty items would you choose to add to the reception area of a geriatric practice?

_____

_____

_____

4. How would the reception areas of a family doctor and an orthopedist be similar, and how would they be different?

_____

_____

_____

5. What could you do to learn more about your office's patients in order to make the reception area more appealing?

_____

_____

_____

APPLICATION

Follow the directions for the application.

Creating a Reception Area

Working with a partner, imagine that you have been asked to create a patient reception area for a small medical office. As you plan the area, keep the needs and comfort of the patients foremost in your minds.

a. With your partner, decide on the kind of practice for which you will be creating a reception area, such as a gerontology, orthopedic, or family practice. Then brainstorm a list of the characteristics, needs, and interests of the patients of this practice. Put the kind of practice and your list in writing.

b. Determine the size of the reception area. Base the size on the number of patients who will be using the reception area at one time. Make a diagram or floor plan of the area. If you wish, use graph paper and draw the area to scale. For example, you might decide that one square on the graph paper equals 2 feet in the reception area. Locate all doors and windows. Draw them to scale on the diagram.

c. Discuss the decor. Choose a color family, and select colors for the carpeting, furniture, walls, window treatments, and so on. Keep written notes of your selections.

d. Decide what furniture you will purchase and how it will be arranged. Keep in mind the needs of the kinds of patients who will use the reception area. Locate each piece of furniture on your diagram of the area, drawing each to scale.

e. Choose music, specific magazines and books, and special items for the reception area. Write down your choices.

f. Along with other pairs of students, share your diagram and written notes with the class. Join in a class discussion of the various reception area plans and how each area will meet the specific needs of the medical practice and its patients.

CASE STUDIES

Write your response to each case study on the lines provided.

Case 1

On your first day as a medical assistant for a pediatrician, you notice that the reception area is littered with toys, food wrappers, and other trash. When you mention the mess to the other medical assistant, he replies, "If you clean it up now, it will be back to the same mess in 20 minutes. I just wait until the end of the day and clean the room once." Is this a problem? If so, what can you do?

_____

_____

_____

Case 2

One patient visits the medical office where you work at least once a week and brings her two preschoolers. At first, she asked you to keep an eye on them while she was in the examining room. Now she just leaves the children in the reception area, expecting you to babysit without being asked. You cannot stay in the reception area and watch her children. How can you handle this problem?

_____

_____

_____

Case 3

A pediatric practice has a small paved area just behind the office. Another medical assistant thinks the space could be used for a basketball court where children who are not sick could play while they wait for the doctor to see them or a sibling. Is this a good idea? Explain.

_____

_____

_____

Case 4

The physician in the practice where you work brings in a coatrack that once belonged to his great-grandparents. He is clearly proud of it. You notice, however, that it leans to one side whenever anyone hangs a coat on it. You are concerned that the coatrack might fall over and injure someone. What can you do?

_____

_____

_____

PROCEDURE COMPETENCY CHECKLISTS

PROCEDURE 13.1   Creating a Pediatric Playroom

This procedure outlines the steps for creating a safe and comfortable playroom for pediatric patients. These steps include choosing appropriate books and toys, grouping furniture effectively, and decorating the area to meet the needs of children.

Name _____ Class _____ Date _____

Complete the steps below. A scoring system has been provided for each procedure. The total score for each individual procedure is 100 points. Each step within the procedure is weighted according to the importance of that step and is noted in the column "Point Value." Steps that are of a more critical nature have been weighted with a higher point value. Record your points for each step in the column "Points Achieved."

Determine your mastery of each step in the procedure by assigning it a score of 1 to 4 in the last column: 1 = poor, 2 = fair, 3 = good, 4 = excellent.

On the basis of your scores, budget time for additional practice of specific steps.

Materials: Children's books and magazines, games, toys, crayons and coloring books, television and videocassette recorder (VCR), children's videotapes, child- and adult-size chairs, child-size table, bookshelf, boxes or shelves, decorative wall hangings or educational posters (optional)

Step	Point Value	Points Achieved	Mastery
1. Place all adult-size and some child-size chairs against the wall.	10		
2. Place the remainder of the child-size chairs in small groupings throughout the room. Put several chairs with the child-size table.	10		
3. Put the books, magazines, crayons, and coloring books on the bookshelf in one corner of the room near a grouping of chairs.	10		
4. Choose toys and games carefully. Avoid toys that encourage active play or that require a large area. Make sure all toys meet safety guidelines. Watch for loose parts or parts that are smaller than a golf ball. Toys should be easy to clean.	30		
5. Place the activities for older children near one grouping of chairs and the games and toys for younger children near another grouping. Keep toys and games in boxes or on shelves.	15		
6. Place the television and VCR high on a shelf or attach it to the wall near the ceiling. Keep videos behind the reception desk, and periodically change the video in the VCR.	15		
7. Decorate the room with wall hangings or posters.	10		

Time limit: 10 minutes   Add Points Achieved: _____

Observer's Name: _____

Steps that require more practice: _____

_____

Instructor comments: _____

_____

_____

PROCEDURE 13.2 Creating a Waiting Room Accessible to Differently Abled Patients

This procedure outlines the steps in creating a waiting area that is safe according to the requirements of the Americans With Disabilities Act and that includes appropriate furniture arrangement and choice of reading materials and other materials.

Complete the steps below. A scoring system has been provided for each procedure. The total score for each individual procedure is 100 points. Each step within the procedure is weighted according to the importance of that step and is noted in the column "Point Value." Steps that are of a more critical nature have been weighted with a higher point value. Record your points for each step in the column "Points Achieved."

Determine your mastery of each step in the procedure by assigning it a score of 1 to 4 in the last column: 1 = poor, 2 = fair, 3 = good, 4 = excellent.

On the basis of your scores, budget time for additional practice of specific steps.

Materials: Chairs, bars or rails, adjustable-height tables, doorway floor coverings, magazine rack, television and VCR, ramps (if needed), large-type and braille magazines

Step	Point Value	Points Achieved	Mastery
1. Arrange chairs, leaving gaps so that substantial space is available for wheelchairs along walls and near other groups of chairs. Make sure chairs can be moved to allow extra room.	5		
2. Remove any obstacles that may interfere with the space needed for a wheelchair to swivel around completely. Remove scatter rugs or carpeting that is not attached to the floor.	15		
3. Position coffee tables at a height that is accessible for people in wheelchairs.	5		
4. Place office reading materials at a height that is accessible to people in wheelchairs.	5		
5. Locate the television and VCR within full view of patients sitting on chairs and in wheelchairs so they do not have to strain their necks to watch.	5		
6. For patients with visual impairment, include reading materials with large type and in braille.	15		
7. For patients who have difficulty walking, make sure bars or rails are attached securely to walls 34 to 38 inches above the floor to accommodate requirements set forth in the Americans With Disabilities Act. Make sure the bars are sturdy enough to provide balance for patients who need it. Bars are most important in entrances and hallways. Consider placing a bar near the receptionist's window for added support as patients check in.	25		

(continued)

Step	Point Value	Points Achieved	Mastery
8. Eliminate metal or wood sills in doorways. Otherwise, securely attach a thin rubber covering to provide a graduated slope. Be sure the covering is attached properly and meets safety standards.	10		
9. Make sure the office has ramp access.	10		
10. Solicit feedback from patients with physical disabilities about the accessibility of the patient reception area. Encourage ideas for improvements. Address any additional needs.	5		

Time limit: 10 minutes   Add Points Achieved: _____

Observer's Name: _____

Steps that require more practice: _____

_____

Instructor comments: _____

_____

_____

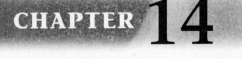

CHAPTER 14

Patient Education

REVIEW

Vocabulary Review

Passage Completion

Study the key terms in the box. Use your textbook to find definitions of terms you do not understand.

consumer education	modeling	philosophy	screening

In the space provided, complete the following passage, using the terms from the box. You may change the form of a term to fit the meaning of the sentence.

Patient education is a vital part of patient care. Preoperative teaching, for example, increases patients' knowledge about and participation in the surgical procedure. Through factual teaching and active demonstrations that include (1) _____, patients learn techniques that can enhance their recovery. (2) _____ that is geared to the average person, in content and in language, helps increase awareness of the importance of good health. This kind of education includes encouraging patients to have regular (3) _____ tests for early diagnosis and treatment of certain diseases. Patients also benefit from learning about the medical office. A statement of (4) _____ in the patient information packet tells them about the values and principles of the practice. Information about office policies and procedures makes patients feel more comfortable with the care they are receiving.

1. _____

2. _____

3. _____

4. _____

Content Review

Multiple Choice

In the space provided, write the letter of the choice that best completes each statement or answers each question.

_____ 1. An important goal of patient education is to
   A. expedite office procedures.
   B. inform the office about staff roles.
   C. enhance the physician's reputation.
   D. promote good health.

_____ 2. Which of the following topics would an educational newsletter most likely contain?
   A. Health-care tips
   B. A physician's credentials
   C. The payment policies of a medical office
   D. A community resource directory

_____ 3. Which of the following tests is *not* an example of a screening test?
   A. A Pap smear
   B. Arthroscopy
   C. A prostate examination
   D. A mammogram

_____ 4. Some practices create simplified versions of their patient information packet for patients
   A. with hearing impairments.
   B. with visual impairments.
   C. who do not understand English.
   D. who will undergo surgical procedures.

_____ 5. When speaking to a patient who wears a hearing aid, it is best to
   A. filter out loud noises.
   B. raise your voice.
   C. speak at a normal level.
   D. speak very slowly.

_____ 6. Which of the following is the best way to verify that a patient with a visual impairment has understood oral instructions for a procedure?
   A. Having the patient repeat the instructions
   B. Having a family member repeat the instructions
   C. Providing the patient with written instructions
   D. Having the patient write the instructions

_____ 7. A useful tool in preoperative education is a(n)
   A. patient information packet.
   B. educational newsletter.
   C. screening test.
   D. anatomical model.

_____ 8. Which of these is the best definition of patient education?
   A. Patient education is the use of visual material to educate a patient.
   B. Patient education is the demonstration of a technique to a patient.
   C. Patient education is the use of verbal instruction to educate a patient.
   D. Any instructions—verbal, written, or demonstrative—that are given to patients are types of patient education.

_____ 9. Patient education is best done
   A. on the first visit, after the physician has seen the patient.
   B. on the first visit, before the physician has seen the patient.
   C. on follow-up visits because the first visit is too stressful for the patient.
   D. anytime you can share meaningful and helpful information with the patient.

_____ **10.** Many accidents happen because people fail to see potential risks. *Potential risks* means
   A. side effects.
   B. situations or things that can cause harm.
   C. preventive measures.
   D. None of the above

_____ **11.** *Preventive measures* means
   A. patient education.
   B. health-promoting behaviors.
   C. screening.
   D. All of the above

_____ **12.** The patient information packet should include
   A. the first bill or invoice.
   B. a description of the practice and an introduction to the office.
   C. medical brochures describing disease processes that relate to the patient's primary medical condition.
   D. All of the above

_____ **13.** The patient confidentiality statement
   A. supplies a place for the patient to sign before any other practice information is released.
   B. is not commonly used in a pediatric practice.
   C. should state that no information from patient files will be released without signed authorization from the patient.
   D. is not usually part of the information packet.

_____ **14.** Patient education is the responsibility of
   A. the entire staff.
   B. the physician.
   C. the nurse.
   D. the medical assistant.

Sentence Completion

In the space provided, write the word or phrase that best completes each sentence.

_____ **15.** When using _____ educational materials, it is helpful to provide corresponding written materials that patients can keep for reference.

_____ **16.** Health is a complex concept that involves the body, _____, emotions, and environment.

_____ **17.** Patients can decrease their chances of getting certain illnesses and diseases by taking _____ measures.

_____ **18.** A patient information packet should identify office staff members according to their _____.

_____ **19.** Elderly patients who have problems with memory should receive detailed _____ instructions.

_____ **20.** Patients who will undergo a surgical procedure must first sign a(n) _____ form.

_____ **21.** A patient's _____ about upcoming surgery can adversely affect her understanding of preoperative instructions.

_____ **22.** Computer resources for current medical information include CD-ROM disks and _____ services.

Short Answer

Write the answer to each question on the lines provided.

23. What are some examples of printed educational materials and visual educational materials?

_____

_____

_____

24. List three ways to achieve good health.

_____

_____

_____

25. List five healthful habits that patients should be encouraged to incorporate into their daily lives.

_____

_____

_____

26. What are three ways that a patient information packet can be helpful to patients? To a medical office?

_____

_____

_____

27. List five types of information that should appear in a patient information packet.

_____

_____

_____

28. When providing information to elderly patients, what are some important points to remember?

_____

_____

_____

29. Describe the benefits of patient education prior to surgery.

_____

_____

_____

30. Identify and describe three types of preoperative teaching.

_____

_____

_____

31. Describe three general sources of patient education materials besides computer resources.

_____

_____

_____

32. List six practices that a medical assistant should use when educating patients with hearing problems.

_____

_____

_____

33. List five tips for preventing injury in the home.

_____

_____

_____

34. List five tips for preventing injury in the workplace.

_____

_____

_____

35. List ten pieces of information to include in a patient's information packet.

_____

_____

_____

36. List the eight steps to developing an education plan for a patient.

_____

_____

_____

37. List the seven warning signs of cancer by spelling out the word CAUTION.

_____

_____

_____

Critical Thinking

Write the answer to each question on the lines provided.

1. What are the advantages of developing a formal, written educational plan for a patient?

_____

_____

_____

2. How might your approach to educating children about healthful habits differ from your approach to teaching adult patients?

_____

_____

_____

3. Give an example of a statement of philosophy that might appear in a patient information packet.

_____

_____

_____

4. When educating patients with special needs, why is it important to be especially sensitive to their individual circumstances?

_____

_____

_____

5. What are some specific ways that family members can be helpful to a patient prior to surgery?

_____

_____

_____

APPLICATION

Follow the directions for the application.

Preparing a Patient Information Packet

Work with a partner to write the following portions of a patient information packet for a fictional medical practice: introduction to the office, description of the practice, introduction to the office staff, office hours, procedures for scheduling and canceling appointments, telephone policy, payment policies, insurance policies, and patient confidentiality statement.

a. Decide on the type of practice to write about. Determine the size of the practice and the number of physicians and other staff members.

b. Reread the description of the contents of a patient information packet. Keep in mind that material in the packet must be written in a clear, straightforward style. Make notes on types of information that will appear in each section of the packet.

c. Decide whether your packet will be a one- or two-page brochure or pamphlet, a multipage booklet, or a folder with several inserts.

d. Determine the order in which information will appear in the packet.

e. On notebook paper, write specific information for each topic.

f. Review and revise the information to ensure that it is clear and complete.

g. Prepare a mock-up of your patient information packet, using sheets of drawing paper and a folder, if you are using one.

h. Copy the information under appropriate headings in the mock-up of your packet. Add illustrations, diagrams, or a map, where appropriate.

i. Share your patient information packet with other pairs in the class. Discuss differences in the packets, and point out elements that are particularly effective or helpful for patients.

j. Help prepare a classroom display of the packets. Invite everyone in the class to view and read the packets.

k. In a full-class discussion, describe the most important points for medical assistants to keep in mind when preparing a patient information packet. Suggest ways to distribute packets to patients.

CASE STUDIES

Write your response to each case study on the lines provided.

Case 1

During a physical examination, a teenage patient admits to you that he lives "mainly on hamburgers and french fries," that he rarely exercises, and that he often gets fewer than 6 hours of sleep a night, except on weekends. "I'll worry about my health when I'm older," he tells you. What can you say to the patient to encourage him to adopt healthful habits now?

_____
_____
_____

Case 2

The physician you work for wants you to develop patient information that will fit on two sides of a 4- by 6-inch index card. There will be room for only the most important information. What should appear on the card?

_____
_____
_____

Case 3

You need to give instructions on the use of medication to a patient who does not speak English. Her son, who has brought her to the medical office, understands English. How will you ensure that the patient fully understands your instructions?

_____
_____
_____

Case 4

A patient calls with questions about her upcoming surgery. Her patient record reflects that the physician has already discussed the nature of the surgery with her. As a medical assistant, what are your responsibilities for ensuring that the patient is fully prepared for the surgery?

_____
_____
_____

PROCEDURE COMPETENCY CHECKLISTS

PROCEDURE 14.1   Developing a Patient Education Plan

This procedure includes identifying the patient's needs; developing a teaching plan; and implementing, evaluating, and revising the plan as indicated.

Name _____ Class _____ Date _____

Complete the steps below. A scoring system has been provided for each procedure. The total score for each individual procedure is 100 points. Each step within the procedure is weighted according to the importance of that step and is noted in the column "Point Value." Steps that are of a more critical nature have been weighted with a higher point value. Record your points for each step in the column "Points Achieved."

Determine your mastery of each step in the procedure by assigning it a score of 1 to 4 in the last column: 1 = poor, 2 = fair, 3 = good, 4 = excellent.

On the basis of your scores, budget time for additional practice of specific steps.

Materials: Pen, paper, various educational aids

Step	Point Value	Points Achieved	Mastery
1. Identify the patient's needs for education. Consider the patient's current knowledge, misconceptions the patient may have, obstacles to learning (loss of hearing or vision, limitations of mobility, language barriers, and so on), the patient's willingness to learn, and how the patient will use the information.	20		
2. Develop and outline a plan using the various educational aids available. Include what you want to accomplish, how you plan to accomplish it, and how you will determine whether the teaching was successful.	10		
3. Write the plan. Try to make the information interesting for the patient.	10		
4. Before carrying out the plan, share it with the physician to get approval and suggestions for improvement.	10		
5. Perform the instruction.	15		
6. Document the teaching in the patient's chart.	15		
7. Evaluate the effectiveness of your teaching session by asking yourself whether you covered all the topics in the plan, whether the information was well received by the patient, whether the patient appeared to learn, and how you would rate your performance.	10		
8. Revise your plan as necessary to make it even more effective.	10		

Time limit: 10 minutes   Add Points Achieved: _____

Observer's Name: _____

Steps that require more practice: _____

_____

Instructor comments: _____

_____

_____

PROCEDURE 14.2   Informing the Patient of Guidelines for Surgery

This procedure includes reviewing the patient's chart, determining the type of procedure, providing appropriate oral and written guidelines for the procedure, and documenting the instructions in the patient's chart.

Complete the steps below. A scoring system has been provided for each procedure. The total score for each individual procedure is 100 points. Each step within the procedure is weighted according to the importance of that step and is noted in the column "Point Value." Steps that are of a more critical nature have been weighted with a higher point value. Record your points for each step in the column "Points Achieved."

Determine your mastery of each step in the procedure by assigning it a score of 1 to 4 in the last column: 1 = poor, 2 = fair, 3 = good, 4 = excellent.

On the basis of your scores, budget time for additional practice of specific steps.

Materials: Patient chart, surgical guidelines

Step	Point Value	Points Achieved	Mastery
1. Review the patient's chart to determine the type of surgery to be performed.	10		
2. Tell the patient that you will be providing both oral and written instructions that should be followed prior to surgery.	5		
3. Inform the patient about policies regarding makeup, jewelry, contact lenses, wigs, dentures, and so on.	10		
4. Tell the patient to leave money and valuables at home.	5		
5. If applicable, suggest appropriate clothing for the patient to wear for postoperative ease and comfort.	5		
6. Explain the need for someone to drive the patient home following an outpatient surgical procedure.	5		
7. Tell the patient the correct time to arrive in the office or at the hospital for the procedure.	10		
8. Inform the patient of dietary restrictions. Use specific, clear instructions about what may or may not be ingested and at what time the patient must abstain from eating or drinking. Explain the reason for the dietary restrictions and the possible consequences of not following them.	10		
9. Ask patients who smoke to refrain from or reduce cigarette smoking during at least the 8 hours prior to the procedure. Explain to the patient that reducing smoking improves the level of oxygen in the blood during surgery.	5		
10. Suggest that the patient shower or bathe the morning of the procedure or the evening before.	5		
11. Instruct the patient about medications to take or avoid before surgery.	10		

(continued)

Step	Point Value	Points Achieved	Mastery
12. If necessary, clarify information about which the patient is unclear.	5		
13. Provide written surgical guidelines, and suggest that the patient call the office if additional questions arise.	5		
14. Document the instruction in the patient's chart.	10		

Time limit: 10 minutes   Add Points Achieved: _____

Observer's Name: _____

Steps that require more practice: _____

_____

Instructor comments: _____

_____

_____

CHAPTER 15

Processing Health-Care Claims

REVIEW

Vocabulary Review

Matching

Match the key terms in the right column with the definitions in the left column by placing the letter of each correct answer in the space provided.

_____ 1. A federally funded health insurance program for Americans aged 65 and older

_____ 2. Payments made by an insurance carrier to a policyholder

_____ 3. An authorization for an insurance carrier to pay a physician or practice directly

_____ 4. The basic annual cost of health-care insurance paid by a policyholder

_____ 5. A fixed percentage of covered charges paid by the insured after the deductible is met

_____ 6. Authorization from a physician for a patient to receive additional services from another physician or medical facility

_____ 7. A managed care organization that creates a specific group of health-care providers from which patients must receive services

_____ 8. A health-care benefit system for families of veterans with total, permanent, service-connected disabilities and for surviving spouses and children of veterans who died in the line of duty

_____ 9. The person in whose name health insurance is carried

_____ 10. An outside service that processes and transmits claims in the correct EDI format

_____ 11. A federally funded health-care benefit system for families of uniformed personnel and retirees from the uniformed services

_____ 12. A form that accompanies payment by an insurer and that can include information about services not covered

_____ 13. Billing a patient for the difference between the physician's charge and the insurance carrier payment

_____ 14. The physician payment structure used by most HMOs

_____ 15. A strategy for keeping health-care costs down by managing, negotiating, and contracting for services

_____ 16. An effort by insurers to prevent duplication of payment for health care

a. assignment of benefits
b. capitation
c. TRICARE
d. CHAMPVA
e. coinsurance
f. coordination of benefits
g. remittance advice (RA)
h. health maintenance organization (HMO)
i. clearinghouse
j. managed care
k. Medicare
l. premium
m. policyholder
n. referral
o. benefits
p. balance billing

Name _____ Class _____ Date _____

True or False

Decide whether each statement is true or false. In the space at the left, write T for true or F for false. On the lines provided, rewrite the false statements to make them true.

_____ 17. A fee-for-service plan repays policyholders for costs for health care.

_____

_____ 18. Some insurers require subscribers to pay a yearly deductible.

_____

_____ 19. According to the birthday rule, the insurance plan of the policyholder whose birthday comes later in the calendar year is the primary payer.

_____

_____ 20. A managed care organization (MCO) sets up agreements with physicians as well as enrolling policyholders.

_____

_____ 21. A fee schedule should be flexible to reflect regional cost differences and differences in physicians' medical education and specialties.

_____

_____ 22. Exclusions are expenses covered by an insurance company.

_____

_____ 23. Eligibility for Medicaid is based on the amount of a patient's reported income for the previous month.

_____

_____ 24. Co-payments are made to insurance companies.

_____

_____ 25. A formulary is a list of excluded prescriptions.

_____

_____ 26. The RBRVS system is the Medicare payment system.

_____

_____ 27. A third-party payer is an insurance carrier.

_____

_____ 28. Preferred provider organizations (PPOs) never allow their members to receive care from providers outside the network.

_____

_____ 29. Medicare Part B has two major programs—Original Medicare Plan and Medicare Advantage.

_____

_____ 30. A lifetime maximum benefit is often established as a total dollar amount by an insurer.

_____

_____ 31. Disability insurance covers the medical expenses of an insured person who is injured or disabled.

_____

_____ **32.** Recipients of Medicare Part A and Part B can purchase Medigap insurance to cover gaps in health insurance coverage.

_____

_____ **33.** The X12 837 Health Care Claim is submitted on paper.

_____

Content Review

Multiple Choice

In the space provided, write the letter of the choice that best completes each statement or answers each question.

_____ **1.** Which of the following tasks is performed by a medical assistant who processes insurance claims?
   A. Filing insurance claims
   B. Writing an explanation of benefits
   C. Collecting premiums from patients
   D. Collecting deductibles from patients

_____ **2.** At the time of service, if required by the health insurance plan, medical assistants collect
   A. deductibles.
   B. co-payments.
   C. premiums.
   D. coinsurance.

_____ **3.** Over half of all health-care plans are
   A. health maintenance organizations (HMOs).
   B. managed care organizations (MCOs).
   C. preferred provider organizations (PPOs).
   D. capitated.

_____ **4.** Under the concept of the resource-based relative value scale (RBRVS) used by Medicare, the fee for a procedure is based on
   A. a combination of the relative value, the geographic adjustment factor, and a conversion factor.
   B. the generally accepted fee that a physician charges for difficult or complicated services.
   C. the average fee that a physician charges for a service or procedure.
   D. the 90th percentile of fees charged for a procedure by similar physicians in the same area.

_____ **5.** The programs offered by TRICARE are
   A. CHAMPUS, TRICARE, and CHAMPVA.
   B. HMO, PPO, POS, and MCO.
   C. TRICARE HMO and TRICARE PPO.
   D. TRICARE Standard, TRICARE Extra, TRICARE Prime, and TRICARE for Life.

_____ **6.** Under Medicare Part B, patients are required to pay an annual
   A. premium.
   B. co-payment.
   C. coinsurance.
   D. claim submission charge for reimbursement.

_____ 7. Coordination of benefits clauses restrict payment by insurance companies to no more than
    A. 150% of the cost of covered benefits.
    B. 100% of the cost of covered benefits.
    C. 90% of the cost of covered benefits.
    D. 80% of the cost of covered benefits.

_____ 8. Patients enrolled in the Original Medicare Plan may purchase additional coverage under a
    A. Medicare Part A plan.
    B. coinsurance plan.
    C. Medigap plan.
    D. Medicare Advantage plan.

Sentence Completion

In the space provided, write the word or phrase that best completes each sentence.

_____ 9. Most employed people have health insurance through _____ **policies.**

_____ 10. An insured's policy can also cover _____ of the subscriber, **such as a** spouse and children.

_____ 11. Some insurers will reject an insurance claim that is not **filed within a** certain _____ limit.

_____ 12. By law, physicians who participate in federally funded **programs such** as Medicare must accept the _____ charge as payment in **full.**

_____ 13. The _____ is the paper claim format.

_____ 14. Patients sign a(n) _____ of benefits statement to **permit providers to** receive payments directly from third-party payers.

_____ 15. Medicare Part A is _____ insurance, whereas Medicare **Part B pays** most of a physician's fee for performing a procedure or **service.**

_____ 16. When filing a Medicaid claim, you should ask for and **check the** patient's Medicaid card to confirm the patient's _____.

_____ 17. Workers' compensation insurance covers accidents or **diseases that are** related to the _____.

Short Answer

Write the answer to each question on the lines provided.

18. List three of the basic steps in the claims process that are performed in a doctor's office.

_____
_____
_____

19. List the three methods of reimbursing physicians that are used by most payers.

_____
_____
_____

20. Describe the process used to calculate what the practice must write off and what a patient owes when the provider is a Medicare participating physician.

_____

_____

_____

21. List three important tips for entering data in billing programs used to prepare health-care claims.

_____

_____

_____

22. Why must the X12 837 Health Care Claim be used for Medicare claims?

_____

_____

_____

23. List three reasons to contact the employer of a workers' compensation patient when the patient contacts the practice for the first time.

_____

_____

_____

24. List the five sections of data elements on the X12 837 Health Care Claim.

_____

_____

_____

25. What three methods are used to submit claims electronically?

_____

_____

_____

Critical Thinking

Write the answer to each question on the lines provided.

1. Why is accuracy important in all aspects of health-care claims processing?

_____

_____

_____

2. For a medical practice, what are some advantages and disadvantages of filing claims for patients rather than having patients pay their medical expenses and file their own claims?

_____

_____

_____

3. Many insurers have had their own claim forms and their own procedures. Why do you think the federal government mandated the HIPAA X12 837 Electronic Claim Transaction that requires the same formats of all payers?

_____

_____

_____

4. Technology known as the "smart card" has been developed to store a person's complete medical history. The information would be easy to access, update, and transmit. Do you foresee any problems with such a system?

_____

_____

_____

5. If you were responsible for processing insurance claims for a medical practice, what aspects of the work do you think you would enjoy most?

_____

_____

_____

APPLICATION

Follow the directions for the application.

Developing Tools for Processing Claims

Work with a partner to analyze the information needed to calculate the practice and patient payments for a new medical practice. The practice will accept patients who have Medicare, Medicaid, workers' compensation insurance, managed care plans, and other types of insurance. The practice will use electronic claims processing.

a. Begin by working with your partner to compile a list of items required for the claims processing steps in your medical office. Include the names of forms (such as the patient registration form); carrier rules (such as time limits); logs; and documents. If you cannot recall the exact name of a publication or form, write a brief description of the information it contains.

b. Review sections of Chapter 15 that describe claims processing for various health plans, such as Medicare, Medicaid, TRICARE and CHAMPVA, Blue Cross and Blue Shield, and PPOs. Add items to the list you began in step a, such as each plan's premium, deductible, coinsurance, and co-payment.

c. Write a brief explanation of how each item is used in processing claims.

d. Identify and list sources of the items, if this information is given in the chapter. If possible, research Web sites for the information using a Web browser.

e. Organize the list by category of items or by type of insurance coverage or benefit on a chart or other type of graphic organizer.

f. Share your chart with other pairs in the class. Discuss various ways to organize these materials in a medical office.

g. In a full-class discussion, analyze the medical assistant's role in handling health-care claims in terms of the procedures and tools needed to comply with current requirements. Discuss ways to reduce the amount of paperwork involved in filing claims. Offer creative suggestions for streamlining or eliminating some steps in the process.

CASE STUDIES

Write your response to each case study on the lines provided.

Case 1

A new patient is completing your office's patient registration form. The patient tells you that she has insurance but does not have her card with her and does not know the effective date of coverage, the group plan number, or the identification number. Explain one or more ways to obtain the insurance information right away.

_____

_____

_____

Case 2

Your medical office receives a payment and a remittance advice (RA) from an insurer in response to a claim you filed for a patient. The RA notes that one of the services on the claim is not covered in the patient's plan. What steps will you take regarding the rejected portion of the claim?

_____

_____

_____

Case 3

As a medical assistant who processes health-care claims for a doctor's office, you make a point of attending local workshops and classes on health insurance and claims processing. A coworker who is learning to file claims says that he does not want to use his free time to attend classes. What could you say to the coworker to try to change his mind?

_____

_____

_____

PROCEDURE COMPETENCY CHECKLIST

PROCEDURE 15.1 Completing the CMS-1500 Claim Form

This procedure outlines the steps involved in completing the CMS-1500 claim form, including obtaining patient information, the patient's signature, clinical information, the charge for services, and the physician's information.

Complete the steps that follow. A scoring system has been provided for each procedure. The total score for each individual procedure is 100 points. Each step within the procedure is weighted according to the importance of that step and is noted in the column "Point Value." Steps that are of a more critical nature have been weighted with a higher point value. Record your points for each step in the column "Points Achieved."

Determine your mastery of each step in the procedure by assigning it a score of 1 to 4 in the last column: 1 = poor, 2 = fair, 3 = good, 4 = excellent.

On the basis of your scores, budget time for additional practice of specific steps.

Materials: Patient medical record, CMS-1500 form, typewriter or computer, patient ledger card

Step	Point Value	Points Achieved	Mastery
Patient Information Section			
1. Check the appropriate insurance box. Enter the insured's insurance identification number as it appears on the insurance card.	5		
2. Enter the patient's name in this order: last name, first name, middle initial (if any).	5		
3. Enter the patient's birth date using two digits each for the month, day, and year. Indicate the sex of the patient.	5		
4. If the insured and the patient are the same person, enter SAME. If not, enter policyholder's name. For CHAMPUS/TRICARE claims, enter the sponsor's (service person's) full name.	2		
5. Enter the patient's mailing address, city, state, and zip code.	3		
6. Enter the patient's relationship to the insured. If they are the same, mark SELF. For CHAMPUS/TRICARE, enter the patient's relationship to the sponsor.	5		
7. Enter the insured's mailing address, city, state, zip code, and telephone number. If this address is the same as the patient's, enter SAME.	3		
8. Indicate the patient's marital, employment, and student status by checking boxes.	2		
9. Enter the last name, first name, and middle initial of any other insured person whose policy might cover the patient. If the claim is for Medicare and the patient has a Medigap policy, enter SAME. 9a. Enter the policy or group number for the other insured person. If this is a Medigap policy, enter MEDIGAP before the policy number. 9b. Enter the date of birth and sex of the other insured person (field 9). 9c. Enter the other insured's employer or school name. (Note: If this is a Medicare claim, enter the claims-processing address for the Medigap insurer from field 9. If this is a Medicaid claim and other insurance is available, note it in fields 1a and 2, and enter the requested policy information. 9d. Enter the other insured's insurance plan or program name. If the plan is Medigap and CMS has assigned it a nine-digit number called PAYERID, enter that number here. On an attached sheet, give the complete mailing address for all other insurance information, and enter the word ATTACHMENT in 10d.	5		

(continued)

Step	Point Value	Points Achieved	Mastery
10. Check the appropriate YES or NO boxes in a, b, and c to indicate whether the patient's place of employment, an auto accident, or other type of accident precipitated the patient's condition. For PLACE, enter the two-letter state postal abbreviation. For Medicaid claims, enter MCD and the Medicaid number at line 10d. For all other claims, enter ATTACHMENT here if there is other insurance information. Be sure the full names and addresses of the other insurer appear on the attached sheet. Also, code the insurer as follows: MSP Medicare Secondary Payer MG Medigap SP Supplemental Employer MCD Medicaid	5		
11. Enter the insured's policy or group number. For Medicare claims, fill out this section only if there is other insurance primary to Medicare; otherwise, enter NONE. **11a.** Enter the insured's date of birth and sex as in field 3, if the insured is not the patient. **11b.** Enter the employer's name or school name here. This information will determine if Medicare is the primary payer. **11c.** Enter the insurance plan or program name. **11d.** Check YES or NO to indicate if there is another health benefit plan. If YES, complete 9a through 9d, or the claim will be denied.	5		
12. Have the patient or an authorized representative sign and date the form here. If a representative signs, have this person indicate the relationship to the patient.	3		
13. Have the insured sign here to authorize payment of Medigap benefits.	3		
Physician Information Section **14.** Enter the date of the current illness, injury, or pregnancy, using eight digits.	2		
15. *Do not complete this field.* Leave it blank for Medicare.	2		
16. Enter the dates that the patient is or was unable to work. This information could signal a workers' compensation claim.	2		
17. Enter the name of the referring physician, clinical laboratory, or other referring source. Enter the physician's unique physician identifier number (UPIN) or other applicable identifying number.	2		
18. Enter the dates the patient was hospitalized, if at all, with the current condition.	2		

(continued)

Step	Point Value	Points Achieved	Mastery
19. Enter the date the patient was last seen by the referring physician or other medical professional.	2		
20. Check YES if a laboratory test was performed outside the physician's office, and enter the test price.	2		
21. Enter the multidigit ICD-9-CM code number diagnosis or nature of injury.	5		
22. Enter the Medicaid resubmission code and original reference number.	2		
23. Enter the prior authorization number if required by the payer.	2		
24A. Enter the date of each service, procedure, or supply provided. 24B. Enter the two-digit place-of-service code. 24C. Leave this field blank. 24D. Enter the CPT/HCPCS codes with modifiers for the procedures, services, or supplies provided. 24E. Enter the diagnosis code that applies to that procedure, as listed in field 21. 24F. Enter the dollar amount of fee charged. 24G. Enter the days or units on which the service was performed, using three digits. 24H. This field is Medicaid specific. 24I. If the service was performed in an emergency room, check this field. 24J. Some plans require a checkmark here if the patient has coverage in addition to the primary plan. 24K. Enter the insurance-company-assigned nine-digit physician PIN. For CHAMPUS/TRICARE, enter the physician's state license number.	5		
25. Enter the physician's or care provider's federal tax identification number or Social Security number.	5		
26. Enter the patient's account number assigned by your office.	2		
27. Check YES to indicate that the physician will accept Medicare or CHAMPUS/TRICARE assignment of benefits.	2		
28. Enter the total charge for the service.	2		
29. Enter the amount already paid by the patient or insurance company.	2		
30. Enter the balance due your office (subtract field 29 from field 28 to obtain this figure).	2		
31. Have the physician or service supplier sign and date the form here.	2		

(continued)

Step	Point Value	Points Achieved	Mastery
32. Enter the name and address of the organization or individual who performed the services.	2		
33. List the billing physician's or supplier's name, address, zip code, and phone number.	2		

Time limit: 10 minutes   Add Points Achieved: _____

Observer's Name: _____

Steps that require more practice: _____

_____

Instructor comments: _____

_____

_____

CHAPTER 16

Medical Coding

REVIEW

Vocabulary Review

Matching

Match the key terms in the right column with the definitions in the left column by placing the letter of each correct answer in the space provided.

_____ 1. A coding reference for medical services performed by physicians

_____ 2. CPT codes used to report the physician's examination of a patient to diagnosis conditions and determine a course of treatment

_____ 3. Acts that take advantage of others for personal gain

_____ 4. CPT codes used to report visits for reasons other than illness or injury

_____ 5. CPT codes used to report procedures done in addition to another procedure

_____ 6. A coding reference for patients' diagnoses

_____ 7. The medically necessary connection between a patient's diagnosis and the procedures performed

_____ 8. A code that is used to report the physician's diagnosis of a patient's condition

_____ 9. A patient who has not received services from the physician within the last 3 years

_____ 10. A list of abbreviations, punctuation guides, symbols, typefaces, and instructional notes that provide guidelines for using a code set

_____ 11. A code set used to report supplies and other procedures on Medicare claims

_____ 12. A code that is used to report the services the physician provided for a patient, such as surgery

a. add-on code
b. code linkage
c. conventions
d. *Current Procedural Terminology* (CPT)
e. diagnosis code
f. E/M code
g. fraud
h. HCPCS Level II code
i. *International Classification of Diseases, Ninth Revision, Clinical Modification* (ICD-9)
j. new patient
k. procedure code
l. V code

True or False

Decide whether each statement is true or false. In the space at the left, write T for true or F for false. On the lines provided, rewrite the false statements to make them true.

_____ **13.** In selecting a code from the ICD-9, you can safely ignore all cross-references.

_____

_____ **14.** A diagnosis is a description of the patient's course of treatment.

_____

_____ **15.** During the global period, follow-up care after a surgical procedure is provided.

_____

_____ **16.** An established patient has seen the physician within the previous three years before this visit.

_____

_____ **17.** A panel is used to group surgical procedures.

_____

_____ **18.** The Alphabetic Index of the ICD-9 is used to verify a code selection after it has been looked up in the Tabular List.

_____

_____ **19.** The Tabular List of the ICD-9 contains codes in numerical order.

_____

_____ **20.** A CPT modifier has three digits and a letter.

_____

_____ **21.** The Health Care Common Procedure Coding System was developed to code workers' compensation claims.

_____

_____ **22.** External causes of accidents and injuries are reported using the ICD-9 E codes.

_____

_____ **23.** Compliance plans represent a process of finding, correcting, and preventing illegal medical office practices.

_____

Content Review

Multiple Choice

In the space provided, write the letter of the choice that best completes each statement or answers each question.

_____ **1.** ICD-9 codes and CPT codes are updated
  A. monthly.
  B. quarterly.
  C. annually.
  D. as needed.

_____ 2. The most specific diagnosis code has
   A. three digits.
   B. four digits.
   C. five digits.
   D. five digits and a modifer.

_____ 3. What type of ICD code is used to report an annual checkup?
   A. V code
   B. E code
   C. Global code
   D. Z code

_____ 4. Where in CPT would you look for guidelines on using each section?
   A. The preface
   B. The notes at the beginning of each section
   C. The appendixes
   D. The descriptions next to each code

_____ 5. The evaluation and management codes in CPT can be used by
   A. only general practitioners.
   B. only dermatologists.
   C. all physicians.
   D. all medical and administrative staff.

_____ 6. Injections and immunizations require two codes, one for giving the injection and second for
   A. the substance.
   B. the E/M.
   C. the V code.
   D. the global period.

_____ 7. In the Health Care Common Procedure Coding System (HCPCS), which codes duplicate the CPT?
   A. Level II
   B. Level I
   C. Category II
   D. Category III

_____ 8. CPT codes are made up of
   A. two digits.
   B. three digits.
   C. four digits.
   D. five digits.

Sentence Completion

In the space provided, write the word or phrase that best completes each sentence.

_____ 9. ICD-9 and CPT are the code sets mandated for _____-compliant health-care claims.

_____ 10. To find the correct ICD-9-CM code, begin by looking up the main term in the Alphabetic _____.

_____ **11.** The codes in the ICD-9's Tabular List are organized according to the source or _____ system.

_____ **12.** A(n) _____ code for accidental poisoning is selected from the ICD-9.

_____ **13.** A _____ is added to the CPT code to show that some special circumstance applied to the service or procedure the physician is reporting.

_____ **14.** Codes in the _____ section of CPT cover all the procedures involved with the operation.

_____ **15.** The next revision of the diagnostic code set is called the ICD-_____-CM.

_____ **16.** Each of the tests in a laboratory _____ should not also be billed separately.

_____ **17.** Billing for procedures that were not done is an example of insurance _____.

Short Answer

Write the answer to each question on the lines provided.

18. List the six sections of the CPT coding reference.

_____
_____
_____

19. List three important conventions in the ICD-9.

_____
_____
_____

20. List the five steps involved with selecting a correct ICD-9-CM code.

_____
_____
_____

21. List the three key factors that determine the level of an evaluation and management (E/M) service.

_____
_____
_____

22. List the five steps involved with selecting a correct CPT code.

_____
_____
_____

Critical Thinking

Write the answer to each question on the lines provided.

1. Why is accurate coding important?

   _____

   _____

   _____

2. How is the medical necessity of the procedures performed for patients demonstrated to **payers?**

   _____

   _____

   _____

3. Why are medical offices advised to keep the previous year's code books?

   _____

   _____

   _____

4. Why should medical practices have a compliance plan?

   _____

   _____

   _____

APPLICATIONS

Follow the directions for each application.

1. **Becoming Familiar with ICD-9-CM**

   Work with a partner. Use the most recent ICD-9-CM reference available to you.

   a. Using Appendix E of the ICD-9-CM, select four of the three-digit disease categories to **study, such** as iron deficiency anemias, chronic pulmonary heart disease, and diabetes mellitus.

   b. Study the entries for the selected category in the Tabular List. Make a note of the **appearance of** any conventions. If a *code also underlying condition* instruction is found, research the **possible** choice.

   c. Prepare a report of the codes that require fourth or fifth digits in each of the **categories.**

2. **Becoming Familiar with CPT**

   Work with a partner. Use the most recent CPT reference available to you.

   a. In the Surgery Section of the CPT, find the heading "Subsection Information" in the **Surgery** Guidelines.

   b. Read the subsection notes for Removal of Skin Tags, Shaving of Lesions, Excision—**Benign Lesions,** and Excision—Malignant Lesions, analyzing the type of instructions provided.

   c. Prepare a comparison table of the instructions of the four subsection notes, **covering these topics:**
      • Definition of Method
      • Type of Anesthesia Covered
      • Use of Lesion Size to Select Code
      • Instructions on Modifiers

CASE STUDIES

Write your response to each case study on the lines provided.

Case 1

A patient presented for evaluation after a fainting spell. The following tests were ordered by the physician: carbon dioxide, chloride, potassium, and sodium. The health-care claim that was submitted contained procedure codes for each test. You have not received any payment on this claim, although payments for other claims sent to the same carrier on that day have been received. What do you think accounts for the delay?

_____

_____

_____

Case 2

A 64-year-old male patient presented for his annual complete physical examination. A routine 12-lead electrocardiogram (ECG) and a general health panel laboratory test were also performed. What procedure codes and diagnosis code would you report on a health-care claim for this service?

_____

_____

_____

Case 3

A patient with acute appendicitis with generalized peritonitis had an appendectomy that was performed using laparoscopy. What procedure code and diagnosis code would you report?

_____

_____

_____

PROCEDURE COMPETENCY CHECKLISTS

PROCEDURE 16.1   Locating an ICD-9-CM Code

This procedure covers the steps involved in finding the appropriate diagnosis codes for use in completing health insurance claim forms.

Complete the steps below. A scoring system has been provided for each procedure. The total score for each individual procedure is 100 points. Each step within the procedure is weighted according to the importance of that step and is noted in the column "Point Value." Steps that are of a more critical nature have been weighted with a higher point value. Record your points for each step in the column "Points Achieved."

Determine your mastery of each step in the procedure by assigning it a score of 1 to 4 in the last column: 1 = poor, 2 = fair, 3 = good, 4 = excellent.

On the basis of your scores, budget time for additional practice of specific steps.

Materials: Patient record, ICD-9-CM

Step	Point Value	Points Achieved	Mastery
1. Locate the statement of the diagnosis in the patient's medical record. This information may be located on the superbill (encounter form) or elsewhere in the patient's chart.	20		
2. Find the diagnosis in the ICD's Alphabetic Index. Look for the condition first. Then find descriptive words that make the condition more specific. Read all cross-references to check all the possibilities for a term and its synonyms.	20		
3. Locate the code from the Alphabetic Index in the ICD's Tabular List. Remember, the number to check is a code number, not a page number. The Tabular List gives codes in numerical order. Look for the number in bold-faced type.	20		
4. Read all information to find the code that corresponds to the patient's specific disease or condition. Study the list of codes and descriptions. Be sure to pick the most specific code available. Check for the symbol that shows that a five-digit code is required.	20		
5. Record the diagnosis code on the insurance claim and proofread the numbers. Enter the correct diagnosis code on the health-care claim, checking the following: • The numbers are entered correctly. Proofread the numbers on the computer screen or on the printed claim form. • The codes are complete. • The highest (most specific) code is used.	20		

Time limit: 10 minutes   Add Points Achieved: _____

Observer's Name: _____

Steps that require more practice: _____

_____

Instructor comments: _____

_____

_____

PROCEDURE 16.2   Locating a CPT Code

This procedure covers the steps involved in finding appropriate procedure codes for use in completing health insurance claim forms.

Complete the steps below. A scoring system has been provided for each procedure. The total score for each individual procedure is 100 points. Each step within the procedure is weighted according to the importance of that step and is noted in the column "Point Value." Steps that are of a more critical nature have been weighted with a higher point value. Record your points for each step in the column "Points Achieved."

Determine your mastery of each step in the procedure by assigning it a score of 1 to 4 in the last column: 1 = poor, 2 = fair, 3 = good, 4 = excellent.

On the basis of your scores, budget time for additional practice of specific steps.

Step	Point Value	Points Achieved	Mastery
1. Become familiar with the CPT. Read the introduction and main section guidelines and notes. For example, look at the guidelines for the Evaluation and Management section. They include definitions of key terms, such as *new patient, established patient, chief complaint, concurrent care,* and *counseling.* The guidelines also explain the way E/M codes should be selected.	20		
2. Find the services listed in the patient's record. Check the patient's record to see which services were performed. For E/M procedures, look for clues as to the extent of history, examination, and decision making that were involved.	20		
3. Look up the procedure code(s). First, pick out a specific procedure or service, organ, or condition. Find the procedure code in the CPT index. Remember, the number in the index is the five-digit code, not a page number. In some cases, the patient's medical record shows an abbreviation, an eponym (a person or place for which a procedure is named), or a synonym.	20		
4. Determine appropriate modifiers. Check section guidelines and Appendix A to choose a modifier if needed to explain a situation involving the procedure being coded, such as difficult work or a discontinued procedure.	20		
5. Record the procedure code(s) on the health-care claim. After the procedure code is verified, it is posted to the health-care claim. The primary procedure—performed for the condition listed as the primary diagnosis—is listed first. Match additional procedures with their corresponding diagnoses.	20		

Time limit: 10 minutes   Add Points Achieved: _____

Observer's Name: _____

Steps that require more practice: _____

_____

Instructor comments: _____

_____

_____

CHAPTER **17**

Patient Billing and Collections

REVIEW

Vocabulary Review

Matching

Match the key terms in the right column with the definitions in the left column by placing the letter of each correct answer in the space provided.

_____ 1. An account with only one charge

_____ 2. An account in which the physician and patient sign an agreement stating that the patient will pay the bill in more than four installments

_____ 3. A written description of the agreed terms of payment

_____ 4. A form that includes the charges for services rendered, an invoice for payment or insurance co-payment, and information for submitting an insurance claim

_____ 5. The process of classifying and reviewing past-due accounts by age from the first date of billing

_____ 6. An arrangement that allows the patient time to pay for services

_____ 7. A law that sets a time limit on when a collection suit on a past-due account can legally be filed

_____ 8. An invoice that contains a reminder that payment is due

_____ 9. The court-decreed right to make decisions about a child's upbringing

_____ 10. A system in which each patient is billed only once a month but spreads the work of billing over the month

_____ 11. An account that is open to charges made occasionally

a. age analysis
b. credit
c. cycle billing
d. disclosure statement
e. legal custody
f. open-book account
g. single-entry account
h. statement
i. statute of limitations
j. superbill
k. written-contract account

True or False

Decide whether each statement is true or false. In the space at the left, write T for true or F for false. On the lines provided, rewrite the false statements to make them true.

_____ 12. Immediate payment from patients brings income into the practice and saves the cost of preparing and mailing bills.

_____

_____ 13. Most physicians prefer to collect payments from patients at the end of each month.

_____

_____ **14.** The one major disadvantage to the use of credit cards in a medical practice is cost.

_____

_____ **15.** Third-party liability refers to the responsibility of the patient's insurance company to pay for certain medical expenses.

_____

_____ **16.** The price list for a medical practice is called a charge slip.

_____

Content Review

Multiple Choice

In the space provided, write the letter of the choice that best completes each statement or answers each question.

_____ **1.** If the patient sues the practice for violation of the Equal Credit Opportunity Act, the practice
  A. is not liable.
  B. may have to pay damages.
  C. may countersue the patient.
  D. None of the above

_____ **2.** A practice may buy accounts receivable insurance to protect the practice from
  A. welfare patients.
  B. employee theft.
  C. lost income because of nonpayment.
  D. malpractice.

_____ **3.** The Fair Debt Collection Practices Act of 1977
  A. allows you to call patients at any time to get payment.
  B. permits you to threaten to turn the account over to collections.
  C. permits you to harass the patient daily for payment.
  D. governs the methods that can be used to collect unpaid debts.

_____ **4.** Free treatment for hardship cases is
  A. up to the receptionist to allow.
  B. expected by all patients in all cases.
  C. at the doctor's discretion.
  D. never permitted.

_____ **5.** To encourage prompt payment from the patient, the practice
  A. calls the patient regularly.
  B. mails reminder letters daily.
  C. insists on payment at time of service.
  D. encloses a stamped envelop with the invoice.

_____ **6.** A hardship case is defined as a person who is
  A. poor.
  B. underinsured.
  C. uninsured.
  D. All of the above

7. The Truth in Lending Act
_____
   A. must be agreed on by the patient and the physician.
   B. covers credit agreements that involve more than six payments.
   C. does not require a disclosure statement.
   D. states that credit agreements cannot be denied.

8. Most practices begin the collection process with
_____
   A. telephone calls, home visits, or letters.
   B. telephone calls, letters, or statements.
   C. credit checks, letters, or statements.
   D. credit checks or collection agencies.

9. Banking tasks in the medical office include
_____
   A. writing checks.
   B. accepting checks.
   C. endorsing checks.
   D. All of the above

Sentence Completion

In the space provided, write the word or phrase that best completes each sentence.

_____ 10. Money paid as punishment for intentionally breaking the law is referred to as _____.

_____ 11. In a class action lawsuit, one or more patients sue a practice that allegedly _____ all of them the same way.

_____ 12. A _____ provides information about the credit worthiness of a person seeking credit.

_____ 13. The use of a _____ for documenting the patient's visit, including diagnosis, procedures, and fees, saves time and paperwork.

_____ 14. Health insurance for dependents of active-duty and retired military personnel is provided by _____.

_____ 15. By law you cannot threaten to send an account to a _____ unless it has not been paid on the stipulated cutoff date.

_____ 16. A _____ is the average fee charged by all comparable doctors in the region.

_____ 17. A quarterly age analysis helps a practice keep on top of _____.

Short Answer

Write the answer to each question on the lines provided.

18. Describe what cycle billing means.

_____

_____

_____

19. What does third-party liability refer to?

_____

_____

_____

20. When determining the responsibilities for minors, the parent who has legal custody can make what type of decisions?

_____

_____

_____

21. What is the definition of the statute of limitations?

_____

_____

_____

22. How would you compute gross collection percentage?

_____

_____

_____

Critical Thinking

Write the answer to each question on the lines provided.

1. A patient is through seeing the doctor, and he hands you his charge slip for services. You ask how he would like to pay. He hands you a credit card that the practice does not accept. What do you say?

_____

_____

_____

2. The patient returns from seeing the doctor and hands you the superbill form on which the doctor has checked services rendered as "comprehensive," but the patient argues that the visit was "limited." How do you handle this situation?

_____

_____

_____

3. When handing a patient's account over to a collection agency, what information should you supply about the patient?

_____

_____

_____

4. Why is it best to be careful in choosing a collection agency?

_____

_____

_____

5. Imagine that the doctor in your office is extending credit to a patient. What are the benefits of extending credit?

_____

_____

_____

APPLICATION

Follow the directions for the application.

Using the knowledge gained in the text, including Chapter 17, design a charge table or form that clearly defines each type of office care. Include such information as (a) is the patient a new patient, (b) is the patient an established patient, (c) was the appointment simply a consultation, (d) did the patient receive limited care, (e) did the patient receive comprehensive care, and so on. Define each type of care in detail so as to avoid any billing questions. A patient may come to you and argue that the type of care she received was "limited" and the physician checked "comprehensive" on the bill. You will need this form to show the patient exactly which services are given under each type of care.

CASE STUDIES

Write your response to each case study on the lines provided.

Case 1

A patient comes to you to pay for his office visit. He hands you the check and says he is in a hurry and cannot wait for a receipt. He leaves, and you notice he has not signed the check. What do you do?

_____

_____

_____

Case 2

You have sent a check to the janitorial service company that cleans your office nightly. The very day that you sent the check, the doctor tells you he is very dissatisfied because the trash in his office has not been emptied all week. You call the company and inform them of your dissatisfaction, but that night the trash is still not emptied. What would you do?

_____

_____

_____

PROCEDURE COMPETENCY CHECKLIST

PROCEDURE 17.1   How to Bill With the Superbill

This procedure outlines the steps involved in using a superbill for patient billing. These steps include completing the physician's name and address, patient information, total charges, patient payments, and the final balance.

Complete the steps below. A scoring system has been provided for each procedure. The total score for each individual procedure is 100 points. Each step within the procedure is weighted according to the importance of that step and is noted in the column "Point Value." Steps that are of a more critical nature have been weighted with a higher point value. Record your points for each step in the column "Points Achieved."

Name _____ Class _____ Date _____

Determine your mastery of each step in the procedure by assigning it a score of 1 to 4 in the last column:
1 = poor, 2 = fair, 3 = good, 4 = excellent.

On the basis of your scores, budget time for additional practice of specific steps.

Materials: Superbill, patient ledger card, patient information sheet, fee schedule, insurance code list, pen

Step	Point Value	Points Achieved	Mastery
1. Make sure the doctor's name and address appear on the form.	5		
2. From the patient ledger card and information sheet, fill in the patient's data, such as name, sex, date of birth, and insurance information.	10		
3. Fill in the place and date of service.	5		
4. Attach the superbill to the patient's medical record, and give them both to the doctor.	5		
5. Accept the completed superbill from the patient after the patient sees the doctor. Make sure that the doctor has indicated the diagnosis and the procedures performed.	15		
6. If the doctor has not already recorded the charges, refer to the fee schedule. Then fill in the charges next to the marked procedures.	10		
7. List the total charges for the visit and the previous balance (if any). Deduct any payments or adjustments received before this visit.	10		
8. Calculate the subtotal.	10		
9. Fill in the amount and type of payment (cash, check, money order, or credit card) made by the patient.	5		
10. Calculate and enter the new balance.	10		
11. Have the patient sign the authorization-and-release section of the superbill.	10		
12. Keep a copy of the superbill. Give the patient the original and a copy to file with the patient's insurer.	5		

Time limit: 10 minutes   Add Points Achieved: _____

Observer's Name: _____

Steps that require more practice: _____

_____

Instructor comments: _____

_____

_____

CHAPTER **18**

Accounting for the Medical Office

REVIEW

Vocabulary Review

Matching

Match the key terms in the right column with the definitions in the left column by placing the letter of each correct answer in the space provided.

_____ 1. A certificate of guaranteed payment that may be purchased from banks, post offices, and some convenience stores

_____ 2. The document prepared for each patient that includes the patient's name, address, home and work telephone numbers, and the name of the person responsible for payment

_____ 3. A bank draft or order for payment

_____ 4. Amounts regularly withheld from your paycheck, such as federal, state, and local taxes

_____ 5. The record that shows the total owed to the practice

_____ 6. A check made out to the patient rather than to the practice

_____ 7. A bookkeeping procedure performed to be sure the office and bank records are consistent

_____ 8. The person who receives the payment

_____ 9. The legal right to handle financial matters for another person who is mentally or physically unable to do so

_____ 10. The process of recording in a daily log each of the following: service provided, fee charged, and payment received

_____ 11. Goods or properties that have a dollar value, such as a medical practice building, bank account, office equipment, and accounts receivable

_____ 12. To write something on the back of a check, such as the doctor's name and "For Deposit Only"

_____ 13. A check issued on bank paper and signed by a bank representative

_____ 14. Cash kept on hand in the office to cover minor expenses

_____ 15. The amount of take-home pay that an employee gets after all deductions are made from gross earnings

_____ 16. A record of the amount of cash available to cover expenses, invest, or take out as profit

a. cashier's check
b. check
c. payee
d. patient ledger card
e. endorse
f. third-party check
g. accounts receivable
h. money order
i. payroll deductions
j. benefits
k. assets
l. reconciliation
m. power of attorney
n. journalizing
o. cash flow statement
p. net earnings
q. petty cash fund

True or False

Decide whether each statement is true or false. In the space at the left, write T for true or F for false. On the lines provided, rewrite the false statements to make them true.

_____ **17.** Medical assistants can obtain information for the daily log from word of mouth from patients.

_____

_____ **18.** An account card is the same thing as a record of office disbursements.

_____

_____ **19.** To help with the practice's bookkeeping and banking, you need to understand basic accounting systems and have certain financial management skills.

_____

_____ **20.** You should record payments for out-of-office visits by recording them only in a separate daily log.

_____

_____ **21.** All bookkeeping systems include records of income, charges (money owed to the practice), and disbursements (money paid out by the practice).

_____

_____ **22.** The ABA number on a check identifies the geographical area and the specific bank on which the check is drawn.

_____

_____ **23.** A check would be non-negotiable if it is signed.

_____

_____ **24.** The purpose of the disbursements log is to provide a record of each patient.

_____

_____ **25.** Information on a patient ledger card includes the patient's name, address, phone number(s), and the name of the person responsible for the charges (if different from the patient).

_____

_____ **26.** After you subtract the petty cash receipts from the original balance in the petty cash fund, the difference should equal the original amount in the fund.

_____

_____ **27.** FICA taxes fund Social Security and Medicare.

_____

Content Review

Multiple Choice

In the space provided, write the letter of the choice that best completes each statement or answers each question.

_____ **1.** The purpose of the daily log is to
   A. provide a record of each patient seen.
   B. list appointments.
   C. reconcile all finances.
   D. None of the above

_____ 2. The pegboard system
         A. is called the one-write system.
         B. records transactions on one form.
         C. is accurate and easy to learn.
         D. All of the above

_____ 3. The patient ledger card does not include the patient's
         A. name.
         B. Social Security number.
         C. driver's license number.
         D. work number.

_____ 4. Payments for out-of-office visits should be recorded by
         A. having the doctor fill out a charge slip or receipt.
         B. recording each payment on the patient ledger card and the daily log.
         C. recording each payment in a separate daily log.
         D. creating a special payment ledger.

_____ 5. The double-entry accounting system is based on the following accounting equation:
         A. Assets = Liabilities + Owner Equity
         B. Assets + Liabilities = Owner Equity
         C. Assets + Owner Equity = Liabilities
         D. None of the above

_____ 6. Most bookkeeping software programs include
         A. grammar and spell-check features.
         B. built-in tax tables.
         C. electronic endorsements.
         D. built-in check codes.

_____ 7. Banking tasks in the medical office include
         A. writing checks.
         B. accepting checks.
         C. endorsing checks.
         D. All of the above

_____ 8. The Fair Labor Standards Act
         A. limits the number of hours that employees may work.
         B. sets limits on minimum wages for employees.
         C. regulates overtime pay for employees.
         D. All of the above

_____ 9. The employee's payroll information sheet
         A. is maintained by the employee.
         B. does not include the employee's hourly wage rate.
         C. must maintain up-to-date, accurate payroll information about each employee.
         D. None of the above

Sentence Completion

In the space provided, write the word or phrase that best completes each sentence.

_____ 10. An accounts payable record shows the amounts the practice owes to _____.

_____ 11. Papers that are _____ are legally transferable from one person to another.

_____ 12. Whereas assets are goods or properties that are part of the worth of a practice, liabilities are amounts owed by the practice to _____.

_____ 13. Both sides of a(n) _____ accounting equation must always balance or agree.

_____ 14. A person who writes a check is known as a _____.

_____ 15. The ABA number on a printed check is a bank identification number that appears in the form of a fraction on the _____ of the check.

_____ 16. A medical assistant receives an additional $40 in her paycheck for a week in which she worked an extra hour every day. This makes her payroll type _____.

_____ 17. When paychecks are deposited _____, employees can withdraw their pay the same day it is deposited.

Short Answer

Write the answer to each question on the lines provided.

18. Describe the importance of accuracy in bookkeeping and banking.

_____

_____

_____

19. In a record of office disbursements, what is the difference between a payee and a payer?

_____

_____

_____

20. What is the advantage of using the pegboard system?

_____

_____

_____

21. Why is it advantageous to make frequent bank deposits?

_____

_____

_____

22. Why is it important to endorse or write a check in ink?

_____

_____

_____

23. What are four things you can find out by telephone banking?

_____

_____

_____

24. How do you start a petty cash fund?

_____

_____

_____

Critical Thinking

Write the answer to each question on the lines provided.

1. What is the purpose of a deposit slip?

_____

_____

_____

2. Why is it important to reconcile the monthly bank statement with your checkbook balance?

_____

_____

_____

3. Name some of the information listed on the patient ledger card and why each is important to keep up-to-date.

_____

_____

_____

4. Why is patience and empathy so important to a patient?

_____

_____

_____

APPLICATION

Follow the directions for the application.

Using a ledger sheet—either one purchased in an office supply store or one made up on the computer—create a record of office disbursements for a one-month period using the following information.

a. For the purposes of this exercise, use November 2004. Remember that you'll need a column for the date, payee, check number, and total amount plus each of the expenses listed here. You decide which check number to begin with.

b. Types of Expenses
- rent
- utilities
- postage
- lab/x-rays
- medical supplies
- office supplies
- wages
- insurance
- taxes
- travel
- miscellaneous

c. Monthly Expenses

Use this information to fill in your office disbursements ledger.
- 11/01 – Payment to La Jolla Property Management for rent, $1700.00.
- 11/01 – Payment to Anderson Janitorial for monthly office cleaning, $850.00.
- 11/01 – Office Depot for fax machine paper, $37.89.
- 11/01 – Pacific Telephone for monthly telephone services, $384.57.
- 11/01 – Pacific Gas Company for monthly gas and electric, $683.84.
- 11/01 – Cash for stamps at the post office, $32.00.
- 11/02 – Uni Lab for blood work, $55.00.
- 11/02 – Harris Medical Supply for general medical supplies, $75.00.
- 11/05 – Medi Quik X-Ray, $32.50.
- 11/06 – Staples Office Supply for general office supplies, $68.24.
- 11/12 – City Laundry (uniforms and towels), $125.00.
- 11/15 – Toni Guzzi (payroll), $76.08.
- 11/15 – Terry Smart (payroll), $89.84.
- 11/15 – Janet Garcia (payroll), $125.00.
- 11/15 – James Smith (payroll), $78.76.
- 11/17 – Toni Guzzi (reimbursement for travel expenses), $12.50.
- 11/20 – Stamps at post office from petty cash, $64.00.
- 11/23 – Medi Quik X-Ray, $35.87.
- 11/25 – World Wide Insurance, $189.00
- 11/30 – IRS, $537.00.

d. Be sure your amounts at the total of your record agree with the amounts in each of the accounts.

CASE STUDIES

Write your response to each case study on the lines provided.

Case 1

You are a senior medical assistant in a physician's office in charge of all the bookkeeping and banking tasks. You decided to take a couple of days off and handed your duties off to a less experienced medical assistant. All she needed to do was make the Friday deposit at the bank, and you were supposed to call her on Friday to be sure it was done. You wake up in the middle of the night and are startled to remember that you forgot to call and help her through the process. What methods would you use to determine if the deposit had been made correctly?

_____

_____

_____

Case 2

Your bank statement has arrived in the mail and along with it is a check from a patient marked "Insufficient Funds." What does this mean, and what do you do now to get paid?

_____

_____

_____

Case 3

Your bank statement has arrived in the mail and the balance from the bank does not agree with the balance in your check register. What do you do?

_____

_____

_____

PROCEDURE COMPETENCY CHECKLISTS

PROCEDURE 18.1   Organizing the Practice's Bookkeeping System

This procedure includes starting a new daily log sheet, updating ledger cards, recording deposits, and preparing a charge summary.

Complete the steps below. A scoring system has been provided for each procedure. The total score for each individual procedure is 100 points. Each step within the procedure is weighted according to the importance of that step and is noted in the column "Point Value." Steps that are of a more critical nature have been weighted with a higher point value. Record your points for each step in the column "Points Achieved."

Determine your mastery of each step in the procedure by assigning it a score of 1 to 4 in the last column: 1 = poor, 2 = fair, 3 = good, 4 = excellent.

On the basis of your scores, budget time for additional practice of specific steps.

Name _____ Class _____ Date _____

Materials: Daily log sheets; patient ledger cards; check register; summaries of charges, receipts, and disbursements

Step	Point Value	Points Achieved	Mastery
1. Using a new daily log sheet, record the name of each new patient seen that day. Also record the relevant charges and payments received.	20		
2. Keep ledger cards for all patients, with each patient's name, address, home and work telephone numbers, insurance company, and person responsible for payment. Update the cards, adjusting the balance after every transaction.	20		
3. Record all deposits in the check register. File the deposit receipt with a detailed listing of checks.	20		
4. When paying bills, enter each check in the register. Include check number, date, payee, and amount.	20		
5. Prepare a summary of charges, receipts, and disbursements every month, quarter, or year. Double-check calculations before posting them to summaries.	20		

Time limit: 10 minutes   Add Points Achieved: _____

Observer's Name: _____

Steps that require more practice: _____
_____

Instructor comments: _____
_____
_____

PROCEDURE 18.2   Making a Bank Deposit

This procedure includes sorting the currency, reviewing and listing checks and money orders, calculating the total deposit, making the deposit, and obtaining a receipt.

Complete the steps below. A scoring system has been provided for each procedure. The total score for each individual procedure is 100 points. Each step within the procedure is weighted according to the importance of that step and is noted in the column "Point Value." Steps that are of a more critical nature have been weighted with a higher point value. Record your points for each step in the column "Points Achieved."

Determine your mastery of each step in the procedure by assigning it a score of 1 to 4 in the last column: 1 = poor, 2 = fair, 3 = good, 4 = excellent.

On the basis of your scores, budget time for additional practice of specific steps.

Name _____ Class _____ Date _____

Materials: Bank deposit slip and items to be deposited, such as checks, cash, and money orders

Step	Point Value	Points Achieved	Mastery
1. Divide the bills, coins, checks, and money orders into separate piles.	5		
2. Sort the bills by denomination; stack them, portrait side up, in the same direction. Total and record the amount on the deposit slip line marked "Currency."	5		
3. If there are enough coins, put them in wrappers. If not, count the coins, and put them in the deposit bag. Total the amount of coins, and record that amount on the deposit slip line marked "Coin."	10		
4. Review all checks and money orders for proper endorsements. List each check on the deposit slip, including the check number and amount. If you do not keep a list of the check writers' names in the office, record this information on the deposit slip also.	20		
5. List each money order on the deposit slip with the notation "money order" or "MO" and name of the writer.	10		
6. Calculate the total deposit, and record it on the slip under "Total." Photocopy the slip for office records.	15		
7. Record the total amount of the deposit in the office checkbook register.	15		
8. If you plan to make the deposit in person, place the currency, coins, checks, and money orders in a deposit bag. Otherwise, put the checks and money orders in a special bank-by-mail envelope, or put all deposit items in an envelope and send it by registered mail.	5		
9. Make the deposit in person or by mail.	5		
10. Obtain a deposit receipt from the bank. File it in the office for use in reconciling the bank statement.	10		

Time limit: 10 minutes   Add Points Achieved: _____

Observer's Name: _____

Steps that require more practice: _____

_____

Instructor comments: _____

_____

_____

PROCEDURE 18.3   Reconciling a Bank Statement

This procedure includes matching the previous closing balance with the new statement balance, checking deposits and returned checks against the bank statement, subtracting outstanding checks from the statement balance, and comparing the checkbook balance with the new bank statement balance.

Complete the steps below. A scoring system has been provided for each procedure. The total score for each individual procedure is 100 points. Each step within the procedure is weighted according to the importance of that step and is noted in the column "Point Value." Steps that are of a more critical nature have been weighted with a higher point value. Record your points for each step in the column "Points Achieved."

Determine your mastery of each step in the procedure by assigning it a score of 1 to 4 in the last column: 1 = poor, 2 = fair, 3 = good, 4 = excellent.

On the basis of your scores, budget time for additional practice of specific steps.

Materials: Previous bank statement, current bank statement, reconciliation worksheet (if not part of the current bank statement), deposit receipts, red pencil, check stubs or checkbook register, returned checks

Step	Point Value	Points Achieved	Mastery
1. Check the closing balance on the previous statement against the opening balance on the new statement to make sure they match. If they do not match, call the bank.	10		
2. Record the closing balance from the new statement on the reconciliation worksheet.	10		
3. Check each deposit receipt against the bank statement. Place a red check mark in the upper right corner of each recorded receipt. Total the deposits that do *not* appear on the statement. Add the total to the closing balance on the reconciliation worksheet.	10		
4. Put the returned checks in numerical order.	10		
5. Compare each returned check with the bank statement, making sure that the amounts agree. Place a red check mark in the upper right corner of each returned check that is recorded on the statement. Also place a check mark on the check stub or check register entry.	10		
6. List each outstanding check on the worksheet. Total these checks; then subtract the total from the bank statement balance.	10		
7. Add interest, if interest was earned.	10		
8. Subtract any service charges, check printing charges, or automatic payments.	10		
9. Compare the new checkbook balance with the new bank statement balance. They should match. If they do not, repeat the process, rechecking all calculations and looking for other possible errors.	10		

(continued)

Name _____ Class _____ Date _____

Step	Point Value	Points Achieved	Mastery
10. If your work is correct and the balances still do not agree, call the bank to determine whether a bank error has been made.	10		

Time limit: 10 minutes   Add Points Achieved: _____

Observer's Name: _____

Steps that require more practice: _____
_____

Instructor comments: _____
_____
_____

PROCEDURE 18.4   Setting Up the Accounts Payable System

This procedure includes setting up the disbursements journal, petty cash record, and payroll register.

Complete the steps below. A scoring system has been provided for each procedure. The total score for each individual procedure is 100 points. Each step within the procedure is weighted according to the importance of that step and is noted in the column "Point Value." Steps that are of a more critical nature have been weighted with a higher point value. Record your points for each step in the column "Points Achieved."

Determine your mastery of each step in the procedure by assigning it a score of 1 to 4 in the last column: 1 = poor, 2 = fair, 3 = good, 4 = excellent.

On the basis of your scores, budget time for additional practice of specific steps.

Materials: Disbursements journal, petty cash record, payroll register, pen

Step	Point Value	Points Achieved	Mastery
Setting Up the Disbursements Journal			
1. Write in column headings for the basic information about each check: date, payee's name, check number, and check amount.	10		
2. Write in column headings for each type of business expense, such as rent and utilities.	5		
3. Write in column headings for deposits and the account balance.	5		
4. Record the data from completed checks under the appropriate column headings.	5		

(continued)

Step	Point Value	Points Achieved	Mastery
Setting Up the Petty Cash Record 1. Write in column headings for the date, transaction number, payee, brief description, amount of transaction, and type of expense.	10		
2. Write in a column heading for the petty cash fund balance.	5		
3. Record the data from petty cash vouchers under the appropriate column headings.	5		
Setting Up the Payroll Register 1. Write in column headings for check number, employee name, earnings to date, hourly rate, hours worked, regular earnings, overtime hours worked, and overtime earnings.	20		
2. Write in column headings for total gross earnings for the pay period and gross taxable earnings.	5		
3. Write in column headings for each deduction. These may include federal income tax, FICA tax, state income tax, local income tax, and various voluntary deductions.	20		
4. Write in a column heading for net earnings.	5		
5. Each time you write payroll checks, record earning and deduction data under the appropriate column headings on the payroll register.	5		

Time limit: 10 minutes   Add Points Achieved: _____

Observer's Name: _____

Steps that require more practice: _____
_____

Instructor comments: _____
_____
_____

PROCEDURE 18.5   Generating Payroll

This procedure includes calculating regular and overtime hours worked by each employee, calculating gross earnings, computing appropriate tax deductions, making out the paychecks, and depositing deductions in a tax liability account.

Complete the steps below. A scoring system has been provided for each procedure. The total score for each individual procedure is 100 points. Each step within the procedure is weighted according to the importance of that step and is noted in the column "Point Value." Steps that are of a more critical nature have been weighted with a higher point value. Record your points for each step in the column "Points Achieved."

Determine your mastery of each step in the procedure by assigning it a score of 1 to 4 in the last column: 1 = poor, 2 = fair, 3 = good, 4 = excellent.

On the basis of your scores, budget time for additional practice of specific steps.

Name _____ Class _____ Date _____

Materials: Employees' time cards, employees' earnings records, payroll register, IRS tax tables, check register

Step	Point Value	Points Achieved	Mastery
1. Calculate the total regular and overtime hours worked on the basis of the employee's time card. Enter totals under the appropriate headings on the payroll register.	10		
2. Check the pay rate on the employee earnings record. Then multiply the hours worked (including any paid vacation or paid holidays) by the rates for regular time and overtime. This yields gross earnings.	10		
3. Enter the gross earnings under the appropriate heading on the payroll register. Subtract any nontaxable benefits.	5		
4. Using IRS tax tables and data on the employee earnings record, determine the amount of federal income tax to withhold on the basis of the employee's marital status and number of exemptions. Compute the amount of FICA tax to withhold for Social Security (6.2%) and Medicare (1.45%).	10		
5. Following state and local procedures, determine the amount of state and local income taxes (if any) to withhold on the basis of the employee's marital status and number of exemptions.	10		
6. Calculate the employer's contributions to FUTA and to the state unemployment fund, if any. Post these amounts to the employer's account.	10		
7. Enter any other required or voluntary deductions.	5		
8. Subtract all deductions from the gross earnings to get the employee's net earnings.	10		
9. Enter the total amount withheld from all employees for FICA under the headings for Social Security and Medicare. (The employer must match these amounts.) Enter other employer contributions under the appropriate headings.	10		
10. Fill out the check stub, including the employee's name, date, pay period, gross earnings, all deductions, and net earnings. Make out the paycheck for the net earnings.	10		
11. Deposit each deduction in a tax liability account.	10		

Time limit: 10 minutes   Add Points Achieved: _____

Observer's Name: _____

Steps that require more practice: _____

_____

Instructor comments: _____

_____

_____

NOTES

NOTES

NOTES

NOTES

NOTES

NOTES

NOTES

NOTES

NOTES

NOTES

NOTES

NOTES